Operative Dic
Surgery

Said Saghieh
Stuart L. Weinstein
Jamal J. Hoballah
Editors

Operative Dictations
in Orthopedic Surgery

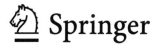 Springer

Editors
Said Saghieh, MD
Division of Orthopaedics
Department of Surgery
American University of Beirut
  Medical Center
Beirut, Lebanon

Stuart L. Weinstein, MD
Department of Orthopedic
  Surgery
University of Iowa Hospitals
  and Clinics
Iowa City, IA, USA

Jamal J. Hoballah, MD, MBA, FACS
Department of Surgery
American University of Beirut
  Medical Center
Beirut, Lebanon

ISBN 978-1-4614-7478-4   ISBN 978-1-4614-7479-1 (eBook)
DOI 10.1007/978-1-4614-7479-1
Springer New York Heidelberg Dordrecht London

Library of Congress Control Number: 2013941474

Springer is part of Springer Science+Business Media (www.springer.com)

Preface

The purpose of this textbook, as any medical publishing, is to enhance our medical practice. We also intend to provide the necessary knowledge to be utilized in a competent medical practice.

The material presented in this book was a thirst to creating a modus operandi for a large majority of surgeries. These modus operandis will serve as guidance for our new clinicians and medical practitioners.

We were motivated to proceed in such an endeavor to facilitate surgical procedures and minimize inquiries and confusion prior to starting surgeries.

Our focus was mostly geared towards setting a model for residents, fellows, and practicing surgeons. These models are templates for practitioners' operative dictations. It also provides the opportunity to compile enough data for the trainee surgeon and gather enough information to participate constructively in the surgery.

This book sheds light on the importance of details in the operating room. These details play a key role in making the surgeons' life easier and enhance the surgical performance. We also wanted to go beyond and specify all detailed preferences, for every particular procedure, crucial for the surgeons.

Our journey, throughout the encrypting of this work, was greatly insightful as it widened our concept of standardization. We have faced numerous procedures, some of which were troublesome and some others that were simple, nevertheless, all of which, allowed the project to be more appealing and fruitful.

Please note that each part of this book describes the most common procedures for an anatomic region.

Different authors contributed to this material and their experience was a definite added-value to this book.

On this note, we extend our acknowledgements to all authors, as they were instrumental in the formation and completion of this book. Their input and participation was necessary and an asset to our writings. Moreover, we shall instill again our appreciation for all those who were devoted to this book and helped us achieve the targeted results.

Beirut, Lebanon	Said Saghieh
IA, USA	Stuart L. Weinstein
Beirut, Lebanon	Jamal J. Hoballah

Contents

Contributors

Ghassan S. Abu-Sittah, MBChB, FRCS Department of Surgery, Plastic and Reconstructive Surgery, American University of Beirut Medical Center, Beirut, Lebanon

Muhyeddine Al-Taki, MD Division of Orthopaedics, Department of Surgery, American University of Beirut Medical Center, Beirut, Lebanon

Bishara Atiyeh, MD, FACS Department of Surgery, Division of Plastic and Reconstructive Surgery, American University of Beirut Medical Center, Beirut, Lebanon

Moustapha Awada, MD Division of Orthopedic Surgery, Department of Surgery, American University of Beirut Medical Center, Beirut, Lebanon

Joseph Bakhach, MD Department of Surgery, Plastic and Reconstructive Surgery, Hand and Microsurgery, American University of Beirut Medical Center, Beirut, Lebanon

John-Erik Bell, MD, MS Department of Orthopaedic Surgery, Dartmouth—Hitchcock Medical Center, Lebanon, NH, USA

Youssef El Bitar, MD Division of Orthopaedic Surgery, Department of Surgery, American University of Beirut Medical Center, Beirut, Lebanon

Saad Dibo, MD Department of Surgery, Plastic and Reconstructive Surgery, American University of Beirut Medical Center, Beirut, Lebanon

Ziad Elkhoury, MD Division of Orthopaedic, Department of Surgery, American University of Beirut Medical Center, Beirut, Lebanon

Erin E. Forest, MD Department of Orthopaedic Surgery, University of California, Davis, Sacramento, CA, USA

Robert Frangie, MD Division of Orthopedic, Department of Surgery, American University of Beirut, Beirut, Lebanon

Geoffrey F. Haft, MD Department of Orthopedic Surgery, Pediatric Orthopedics, Sanford Clinic, Sioux Falls, SD, USA

Mark L. Hagy, MD Department of Orthopaedic Surgery, University of Iowa, University Heights, IA, USA; Lewis Gale Hospital, Virginia Orthopaedic, LLC, Salem, VA, USA

Michael J. Huang, MD Colorado Springs Orthopaedic Group, Colorado Springs, CO, USA

Rida Adel Kassim, MD Division of Orthopaedics, Department of Surgery, Sahel General Hospital, Beirut, Lebanon; Division of Orthopaedics, Department of Surgery, Clemenceau Medical Center, Beirut, Lebanon

Firas Kawtharani, MD Division of Orthopedic Surgery, Department of Surgery, American University of Beirut, Beirut, Lebanon

Aru El Khatib, MD Division of Plastic and Reconstructive Surgery, Department of Surgery, American University of Beirut, Beirut, Lebanon

Joseph G. Khoury, MD Division of Orthopedic Surgery, Department of Surgery, University of Alabama, AL, USA

Karim Masrouha, MD Division of Orthopaedic, Department of Surgery, American University of Beirut Medical Center, Beirut, Lebanon

Anthony V. Mollano, MD Hand and Microvascular Surgery, Concord Orthopaedics PA, Concord, NH, USA

Marc Najjar, MD Division of Orthopedics, Department of Surgery, American University of Beirut Medical Center, Beirut, Lebanon

Rola H. Rashid, MD Department of Orthopaedics, Rochester General Hospital, Rochester, NY, USA

Bernard H. Sagherian, MD Division of Orthopaedic Surgery, Department of Surgery, American University of Beirut Medical Center, Beirut, Lebanon

Said Saghieh, MD Division of Orthopaedics, Department of Surgery American University of Beirut Medical Center, Beirut, Lebanon

Ali Shamseddeen, MD Division of Orthopaedic Surgery, Department of Surgery, American University of Beirut Medical Center, Beirut, Lebanon

Hamdi G. Sukkarieh, MD Division of Orthopedic Surgery, Department of Surgery, American University of Beirut Medical Center, Beirut, Lebanon

Abdel Majid Sheikh Taha, MD Division of Orthopaedics, Department of Surgery, American University of Beirut Medical Center, Beirut, Lebanon

Stuart L. Weinstein, MD Department of Orthopedic Surgery, University of Iowa Hospitals and Clinics, Iowa City, IA, USA

Brian R. Wolf, MD, MS Department of Orthopaedics and Rehabilitation, University of Iowa Hospitals and Clinics, Iowa City, IA, USA

Part I
Pediatrics

Chapter 1

Posterior Spinal Fusion with Instrumentation

Stuart L. Weinstein, M.D.

DIAGNOSIS

Adolescent idiopathic scoliosis

COMMON INDICATIONS

- Progressive scoliosis (Failure of brace treatment).
- Curve greater than 45°.
- Curve greater than 45° with pain unresponsive to nonoperative measures.

POSSIBLE COMPLICATIONS

- Nonunion
- Pseudarthrosis
- Hardware failure
- Neurologic injury
- Transfusion-related risks

ESSENTIAL STEPS

1. Positioning
2. Prepping
3. Skin incision
4. Identification of spinal levels with x-ray or fluoroscopy
5. Subperiosteal dissection of the intended fusion area
6. Obliteration of facet joints
7. Preparation of hook and/or screw sites
8. Measurement of rod

S. Saghieh et al. (eds.), *Operative Dictations in Orthopedic Surgery*,
DOI 10.1007/978-1-4614-7479-1_1,
© Springer Science+Business Media New York 2013

9. Appropriate contouring of rod
10. Exposure of the iliac crest bone graft site
11. Graft harvest
12. Closure of crest site
13. Insertion of rods into hooks and/or screws and correction of deformity
14. Wake-up test
15. Further decortication of spine
16. Placement of bone graft
17. Thoracoplasty if indicated
18. Closure of wound

OPERATIVE NOTE
Preoperative Diagnosis: Adolescent idiopathic scoliosis
Procedure: Posterior spinal fusion with instrumentation
Postoperative Diagnosis: Same
Description of Operation: The patient was taken to the Operating Room. After adequate general anesthesia, he/she was placed prone on the Jackson table (Hall-Relton frame, spine frame, etc.). The arms were abducted 20° and elbows flexed 110° on the arm boards, which were well padded. The iliac crest and breast regions were well padded. The shoulders and upper arms were free. The knees were padded. All bony prominences were checked to make sure they were well protected. Foam pads were placed between the legs and around the legs to prevent bony contact with the OR table. A Bear hugger was used underneath the operating table to maintain the patient's temperature. A second Bear hugger was used on the patient with an opening for the surgical incision. The back was given a two-stage prep and draped free in the usual manner.

A midline incision was made from approximately T1 to L4 and infiltrated with 1:500,000 Epinephrine. Dissection was carried down to the subcutaneous tissues and then down to the spinous processes. A check x-ray was taken to identify levels. The spinous processes were incised with coagulation cautery from T2 to L3. The laminae were exposed subperiosteally to the base of the spinous processes from T2 to L3. The spine was exposed to the tip of the transverse process using Cobb elevators and cautery from the tip of T2 to the tip of L3, taking great care to preserve T1–2 and L3–4 facet joints not to be included in the fusion. All facet joints were cleared of soft tissues. The interspinous ligaments were also removed with a rongeur.

The following was the hook/screw placement pattern:
T2 on the left supralaminar narrow bladed laminar hook.
T2 on the right upgoing pedicle hook.

T3 on the left upgoing pedicle hook.

T4 on the right supralaminar reduced distance laminar hook.

T5 on the left upgoing pedicle hook.

T7 on the right upgoing pedicle hook.

T9 on the left supralaminar reduced distance laminar hook.

T10 on the right upgoing pedicle hook.

T11 on the left supralaminar reduced distance laminar hook.

T12 on the left supralaminar reduced distance laminar hook.

Pedicle screw was placed at L1 on the right 40 mm in length, 5 mm in diameter.

Pedicle screw was placed at L1 on the left 40 mm in length, 6 mm in diameter.

Pedicle screw was placed at L2 on the left 40 mm in length, 6 mm in diameter.

Pedicle screw was placed at L3 on the right 40 mm in length, 6 mm in diameter.

Pedicle screw was placed at L3 on the left 40 mm in length, 6 mm in diameter.

The hooks were secured in the following manner: Pedicle hooks were placed by curettage of the facet joint, squaring off the inferior facet, entering the facet joint with a pedicle finder, and inserting the hook. The supralaminar hooks were placed by curettage of the ligamentum flavum to the superior border of the lamina entering into the spinal canal either with the angled curette or with a nerve hook. The ligamentum flavum was removed or portions of it were removed with the Harper rongeur, and the superior lamina was squared off to allow placement of the hook. The infralaminar hooks were placed by curettage of the soft tissues above the ligamentum flavum, using the laminar elevator underneath the inferior border of the lamina and superior to the ligamentum flavum. If used pedicle screws were placed by identification of pedicles under fluoroscopy, burring out the cortex over the pedicle, sounding the pedicle with the pedicle blunt tipped probe, checking depth position on AP and lateral fluoro picture, tapping the hole to the approximated depth, checking for any penetration of pedicle, and inserting the screw.

Attention was turned to the right iliac crest region. An incision was made 1.5 cm lateral to the posterosuperior iliac spine parallel to the spine incision. The incision extended from the superior aspect of the crest to the notch region. Dissection was carried through the skin and subcutaneous tissues to the gluteal origins. The gluteal muscle origins were incised with coagulation cautery and from 1 cm lateral to the posterosuperior spine to just inferior to the posteroinferior spine. The outer table was removed by the use of osteotomes with one cut 1 cm proximal to the sciatic notch, and the other cuts paralleling the iliac crest. Once the outer table was removed, the medullary contents were removed in cancellous strips by the use of Piggot and Capener gouges. When the majority of the cancellous bone was removed, a ring curette was used to remove more strips of cancellous bone down to the inner table. Finally, a spoon curette was used to remove any remnants of cancellous bone.

The wound was irrigated with copious amounts of saline and packed with thrombin-soaked Gelfoam until the end of the procedure when the gluteal muscles were reattached with running 0 Vicryl. There was no violation of the SI joint or the sciatic notch.

The left rod was measured, cut, and contoured for appropriate sagittal balance. The left-sided rod was inserted into the open hooks and/or screws which were converted to closed hooks by the use of the appropriate closure device. With manual correction of the apex of the thoracolumbar curve, gradual correction was obtained. The rod was fixed proximally and distally, and then the center of the spine was brought to the hooks gradually. Distraction and compression were applied in the appropriate fashion to gain maximal correction, making certain that all hooks maintained good purchase position.

Following this, the right-sided rod was measured, cut, and contoured. It was placed in the open hooks and screws, which were closed with the appropriate closure device. Curve correction was further obtained as per preoperative planning by appropriate compression or distraction.

Motor and sensory monitoring was normal. A wake-up test was completed after maximal correction was obtained and was normal. Two cross-links were applied, both distal to the proximal hooks and proximal to the distal fixation points. All locking mechanisms were secured maximally. All fixation elements were rechecked for purchase and fixation.

The wound and the crest wound were irrigated with copious amounts of saline and Neomycin. The lateral gutters were decorticated and packed with cancellous bone followed by cortical bone, both obtained from the iliac crest. The deep tissues were closed with running 0 Vicryl and the subcutaneous tissues with 2-0 Vicryl over a medium Hemovac. The skin was closed with subcuticular 3-0 Monocryl. The wound was dressed with Steri-strips, Xeroform, Benzoin, and Elastoplast.

Sponge counts were correct.
The patient was taken to the PICU in good condition.
No intraoperative complications.
Staff was present and scrubbed for entire procedure.

Chapter 2

In Situ Fusion L5 to S1

Stuart L. Weinstein, M.D.

DIAGNOSIS
Spondylolisthesis

COMMON INDICATIONS
- In symptomatic low grade Spondylolysis and listhesis of less than 30 %
- Pain unresponsive to nonsurgical methods
- Slip greater than 30–50 % in an immature child

POSSIBLE COMPLICATIONS
- Nonunion
- Cluneal nerve injury
- Infection

ESSENTIAL STEPS
1. Positioning.
2. Prepping and draping.
3. Skin incision.
4. Paraspinous muscle separation.
5. Exposure L5–S1 facet joints.
6. Exposure L5 transverse process and sacral ala.
7. Exposure iliac crest bone graft site.
8. Bone graft harvest.
9. Removal of L5–S1 facet joint.
10. Decortication L5 transverse process, sacral ala, and exposed lamina.

S. Saghieh et al. (eds.), *Operative Dictations in Orthopedic Surgery*,
DOI 10.1007/978-1-4614-7479-1_2,
© Springer Science+Business Media New York 2013

11. Bone graft placement in the facet joint and between the transverse process of L5 and the sacral ala.
12. Closure.

OPERATIVE NOTE

Preoperative Diagnosis: Spondylolysis L5–S1
Procedure: In situ posterolateral fusion L5–S1, iliac crest bone graft
Postoperative Diagnosis: Same
Description of Operation: The patient is taken to the Operating Room and after adequate general anesthesia, is placed prone on a four poster frame (Hall-Relton frame, Jackson table, etc.) with padding under the iliac crest and breast regions. Arms are abducted 20° and elbows flexed 110°. Padding was placed under the down legs and under the down arms. All bony prominences were well padded. The back was given a standard prep and draped free in the usual sterile manner.

A midline incision was made from L4 to S1. The incision was infiltrated with 1/500,000 epinephrine. Dissection was carried down through the subcutaneous tissues, down to the spinous processes of L4–S1. The skin and subcutaneous tissues were elevated off the lumbodorsal fascia approximately 2.5 cm to the right and left side of the midline. On the right side the subcutaneous tissues were also elevated to expose the right iliac crest region. Two hockey-stick incisions were made from the region of approximately the L4 spinous process, carried distally, and then medially toward the S1 spinous process. Each incision was made approximately 1.5–2 cm lateral to the midline. Finger dissection was used to dissect through the paraspinous muscles in a proximal to distal fashion. The L5–S1 joint was palpated through the incision and marked with a Keith needle. A check X-ray was taken to document the appropriate level. The paraspinous muscles were dissected bluntly up to the facet joint of L4–5 taking great care not to injure the capsule at the L4–5 joint. Using a Cobb elevator and bipolar and monopolar cautery, the L5–S1 facet joint was sharply incised and the capsule and soft tissues removed from the facet joint. The ala of the sacrum is exposed subperiosteally with a Cobb elevator, cauterizing all bleeders. The lamina and pars interarticularis defect ["or elongation"] was exposed subperiosteally with a Cobb elevator and/or with judicious use of cautery. The L5 transverse process was palpated and exposed subperiosteally from the base of the lateral aspect of the superior facet joint of L5, taking great care not to injure the capsule of the L4–5 facet joint. The same exposure was accomplished on both the right and left side.

All soft tissues were curetted free from the pars interarticularis defect with a fine curette. The skin and subcutaneous tissues were elevated on the right side with a Hibbs retractor to expose the posterosuperior iliac crest. The gluteal muscles from approximately 2.5 cm superolateral to the posterosuperior spine were incised with coagulation cautery. The incision with cautery was carried along the iliac crest to the posterosuperior and the posteroinferior spine. The outer table of the ilium was exposed subperiosteally. A Taylor retractor was placed into position in the superior aspect of the crest. This allowed exposure of the remainder of the iliac crest. Using a Cobb elevator, the periosteum was gently elevated off the outer table of the ilium down to the level of the sciatic notch. A second Taylor retractor was placed into position to allow complete exposure of the posterior aspect of the iliac crest. Osteotomes are used to remove the outer table of the ilium. This is done by first osteotomizing along the superior aspect of the crest from the posteroinferior spine to the posterosuperior spine of the iliac crest and then carrying the osteotomy along the superior aspect of the crest to the end of the incision. A second osteotomy cut was made approximately 1.5 cm proximal to the sciatic notch and carried approximately three quarters of the way across the crest. The outer table is then removed with straight and curved osteotomes. When the conjoined portion of the ilium is reached, a curved osteotome is used to detach the outer table fragment from the remainder of the crest. The medullary contents are removed by use of Piggott gouges, Capener gouges, ring curettes, and/or spoon curettes taking great care not to enter the sciatic notch or to injure the SI joint. Once all bone graft has been harvested, all bone bleeders were either cauterized or waxed off using bone wax. The wound was packed with thrombin-soaked Gelfoam until the end of the procedure.

Attention was then turned to the spine. The transverse process, sacral ala, and L5 lamina were decorticated using a dental burr. The cancellous bone graft was packed into the 5–1 facet joint, along the lamina and between the L5 transverse process and the ala of the sacrum. A small notch was made in the ala of the sacrum placing bone graft within this notch and anterior to the transverse process of L5 taking great care not to injure the nerve root just anterior to the transverse process. The remainder of the cancellous bone is packed in the lateral gutter, between the transverse process of L5 and the ala. This was followed by packing of the same area with cortical bone. The same procedure is done on both sides.

The wound was then irrigated with copious amounts of saline and antibiotic solution. The Gelfoam was removed from the iliac crest wound, and the wound was irrigated with copious amounts of saline and antibiotic solution. The gluteal muscles were reattached running 0 Vicryl sutures. The lumbodorsal fascia was repaired with running 0 Vicryl. The subcutaneous tissues were closed with 2-0 Vicryl over a medium Hemovac and the skin was closed with a subcuticular 3-0 Monocryl. The wound was dressed with Steri-strips, Xeroform or Adaptic, 4x4's, and a tape dressing.

Sponge counts were correct.

The patient was extubated and taken to the postoperative recovery room in good conditions.

No intraoperative complications.

Staff was present and scrubbed for entire procedure.

Chapter 3

Open Reduction of DDH (Medial Approach)

Joseph G. Khoury, M.D.

COMMON INDICATIONS
- Failure to obtain concentric reduction by closed methods in a child under 12 months of age.

POSSIBLE COMPLICATIONS
- Injury to the obturator nerve.
- Injury to the femoral artery, vein, or nerve.
- Avascular necrosis/deformity of the femoral head.

ESSENTIAL STEPS
1. Transverse incision parallel and just distal to the groin crease
2. Adductor longus tenotomy
3. Develop the interval between pectineus and the adductor brevis
4. Pull the iliopsoas tendon into the wound with a right angled clamp and divide it
5. Identify the capsule and divide it inferiorly around the neck
6. Divide the transverse acetabular ligament and remove any redundant ligamentum teres
7. Remove pulvinar fat
8. Reduce the hip and range it to determine stable position for casting
9. Close wound in standard fashion and apply one and one-half spica cast

S. Saghieh et al. (eds.), *Operative Dictations in Orthopedic Surgery*,
DOI 10.1007/978-1-4614-7479-1_3,
© Springer Science+Business Media New York 2013

OPERATIVE NOTE

Preoperative Diagnosis: Unreducible developmental dislocation of the hip

Procedure: Open reduction and casting

Postoperative Diagnosis: Same

Indications: This 6-month-old child presented late with a uni-lateral dislocation of the hip. Attempts at closed reduction under general anesthetic were not successful. After discussion with the parents, the decision to proceed with open reduction was made.

Description of Operation: The patient was brought to the operating room and positioned supine on the table. After general anesthetic, prepping and draping of the involved lower extremity and the flank were performed in the usual fashion. IV antibiotics were administered.

The patient was secured in the frog leg position.

A 5–7 cm transverse skin incision centered over the anterior margin of the adductor longus, parallel and 1 cm inferior to the inguinal crease was performed.

The adductor fascia was divided longitudinally and the adductor longus was divided close to its origin and retracted distally. The interval between the adductor brevis and the pectineus was developed taking care to avoid damage to the branches of the medial circumflex artery. The iliopsoas tendon was identified, its sheath opened, and the tendon sharply divided and allowed to retract distally.

Next, we attempted a closed reduction and arthrogram. We were not able to obtain an acceptable reduction and continued the operation with an open reduction. The hip capsule was identified and divided. The transverse acetabular ligament divided. The ligamentum teres was divided off the femoral head and acetabulum sharply. A rongeur was used to remove the pulvinar fat. At this point, the hip was easily reduced. Stability was checked. The capsule was closed with 0 Tycron suture.

The wound was irrigated with saline and the hemostasis was achieved. The subcutaneous tissue was closed with vicryl 3-0 and the skin with monocryl 4-0.

Sponge count was correct.

A one and one-half spica cast was applied with the hip in 110' of flexion, 30' of abduction, and 20' of internal rotation.

The patient was extubated and taken to the postoperative recovery room in good conditions.

No intraoperative complications.

Chapter 4
Salter Innominate Osteotomy

Stuart L. Weinstein, M.D.

DIAGNOSIS
Residual hip dysplasia

COMMON INDICATIONS
- Residual hip dysplasia requiring at least 15° of lateral and 25° of anterior coverage.

POSSIBLE COMPLICATIONS
- Infection
- Nonunion
- Pin breakage
- Skin penetration of Steinmann pins
- Damage to the growth of the iliac crest
- Injury to the lateral femoral cutaneous nerve

ESSENTIAL STEPS
1. Positioning
2. Prepping
3. Skin incision
4. Identification of lateral femoral cutaneous nerve
5. Exposure of the iliac crest
6. Exposure of the rectus femoris and hip capsule
7. Over the brim release of the psoas tendon
8. Placement of retractors in the sciatic notch internally and externally
9. Passage of Gigli saw
10. Osteotomy
11. Sectioning of bone graft from iliac crest
12. Placement of graft

S. Saghieh et al. (eds.), *Operative Dictations in Orthopedic Surgery*,
DOI 10.1007/978-1-4614-7479-1_4,
© Springer Science+Business Media New York 2013

13. Figure 4 maneuver to open osteotomy
14. Stabilizing upper fragment of the ilium
15. Insertion of stabilizing pins
16. Wound closure
17. Casting

OPERATIVE NOTE

Preoperative Diagnosis: Residual hip dysplasia

Procedure: Salter innominate osteotomy

Postoperative Diagnosis: Same

Description of Operation: The patient was taken to the Operating Room and after adequate general anesthesia. The involved hip was elevated off of the operating table by placing a (rolled bath blanket, sand bag, or IV bag) underneath the back. The opposite leg and peroneal nerve are protected by foam padding. The entire extremity from the toes to the groin up to the nipple line on the involved side are prepped and draped free in the usual sterile manner. A "bikini" incision is made just below the iliac crest region, extending 3.5 cm proximal to the anterosuperior spine and 1.5 cm distally. Dissection is carried down to the subcutaneous tissues down to the anterosuperior spine. The lateral femoral cutaneous nerve is isolated and protected. The interval between the tensor fasciae latae and the sartorius is identified and developed, taking great care not to injure the lateral femoral cutaneous nerve. The rectus femoris tendon is isolated and dissected free using blunt dissection. Two retractors are placed in the interval between the sartorius and tensor fasciae latae. Placing the thumb and index finger over the iliac crest, the abdominal musculature is moved proximally. Using the index finger with the crest held between the index finger and thumb, the iliac apophysis is incised sharply from the anterosuperior spine posteriorly to approximately the mid crest region. Then the cartilage is incised from the anterosuperior spine directly into the anteroinferior spine. Using Cobb elevators, the apophysis is "popped" off the medial and lateral aspect of the crest. Subperiosteal dissection is used to expose both the inner and outer table of the ilium. The sciatic notch is carefully exposed on the inner table of the ilium using a small Cobb elevator, taking great care not to injure the periosteum and vessels in the sciatic notch. A Cobra blunt tipped retractor was placed in the sciatic notch from the medial aspect. Subperiosteal dissection using a Cobb elevator was also done on the outside of the crest down to the hip capsule and posteriorly into the sciatic notch. A second blunt tipped Cobra retractor is placed into the outer aspect of the sciatic notch. A long curved hemostat is placed in the sciatic notch above the Cobra retractor from medially to laterally. At this point in time, the tendon of the iliopsoas is palpated over the superior brim of the pelvis. Blunt scissor dissection is used to separate the fascia from the tendon. The tendon is exposed and grasped with a curved hemostat and sectioned sharply over the brim of the pelvis.

The Gigli saw is passed into the open tips of the curved hemostat and then the saw is passed from lateral to medial by pushing the saw blade into the notch and pulling using the curved hemostat, taking great care not to initiate the osteotomy cut during the passage of the Gigli saw. Once the Gigli saw has been passed through the notch, the handles are placed and the osteotomy is accomplished by bringing the saw from the notch to the anteroinferior spine taking great care to protect the wound skin edges. Using a large bone cutter, a wedge of bone is removed from the anterior aspect of the iliac crest, approximately 1 cm above the osteotomy in an oblique fashion to include approximately the anterior quarter of the iliac crest. This graft is then fashioned into a wedge. A towel clip is then used to stabilize the proximal portion of the ilium (in the case described, an open reduction is not being accomplished at the same time). The upper section of the ilium is grasped with a towel clip to stabilize the pelvis. The foot of the involved side is placed on the opposite knee is a figure 4 position, pushing down on the knee and pulling the heel toward the patient's chin. This allows opening of the osteotomy in the appropriate line of pull. The distal fragment is grasped with a large towel clip and pulled forward to be certain that it is not displaced posteriorly. The bone graft is then tailored to fit the gap that has been created and is inserted using a Kocher hemostat to grasp the bone graft securely. After the graft has been placed, the sciatic notch is palpated to make certain that the fragment is not displaced posteriorly into the notch. Two heavy threaded Kirschner wires are used to stabilize the fragment passing from the proximal iliac fragment through the bone graft into the distal fragment in a medial and posterior direction. The position of the wires is checked on fluoroscopy and hip range of motion is also checked to be certain that the wires are not inside the hip joint. The wound is then irrigated with copious amounts of saline and antibiotic solution. The iliac apophysis is resecured with interrupted 0 Vicryl sutures. The pins are cut off to protrude just beyond the iliac crest. The two pins are cut at slightly different levels by approximately 1 cm to facilitate later removal. The subcutaneous tissues are closed with 2-0 Vicryl and the skin is closed with subcuticular 3-0 Monocryl. The wound is dressed with Steri-strips, and a Bioclusive dressing or a standard sterile dressing. The patient is then placed in a well-padded 1½ hip spica cast and taken to the postoperative recovery room.

Chapter 5
Pemberton Osteotomy

Stuart L. Weinstein, M.D.

DIAGNOSIS

Hip Dysplasia

COMMON INDICATIONS

- Anterior and/or superolateral acetabular walls deficiency in a child between 2 and 6 years of age.

POSSIBLE COMPLICATIONS

- Infection
- Injury of the lateral femoral cutaneous nerve
- Residual femoral head uncoverage
- Growth arrest and closure of the triradiate cartilage
- Cast sores

ESSENTIAL STEPS

1. Preoperative planning
2. Positioning
3. Identification of lateral femoral cutaneous nerve
4. Identification of the rectus femoris and hip capsule
5. Identification of the sciatic notch
6. Sectioning of the psoas over the pelvic brim
7. Marking with an osteotome of the line of the appropriate osteotomy
8. Osteotomy
9. Opening of the osteotomy
10. Fashioning and placement of the bone graft
11. Closure
12. Casting

S. Saghieh et al. (eds.), *Operative Dictations in Orthopedic Surgery*,
DOI 10.1007/978-1-4614-7479-1_5,
© Springer Science+Business Media New York 2013

OPERATIVE NOTE

Preoperative Diagnosis: Residual hip dysplasia

Procedure: Pemberton osteotomy

Postoperative Diagnosis: Same

Indications: Patient is a ---- old b/g who presented with hip dysplasia.

Description of Operation: The patient was identified and the extremity marked in the preoperative holding area. He/she was brought into the operative suite and placed supine on a radiolucent operating table. The patient was induced into general endotracheal anesthesia without difficulty. IV antibiotics were administered.

The involved hip was elevated off of the operating table by placing a (rolled bath blanket, sand bag, or IV bag) underneath the back. The opposite leg and peroneal nerve were protected by foam padding. The skin of the affected side of the abdomen, pelvis, and the entire lower extremity was prepped and draped in the usual sterile manner.

A "bikini" incision was made just below the iliac crest region, extending 3.5 cm proximal to the anterosuperior spine and 1.5 cm distally. Dissection was carried down to the subcutaneous tissue. The anterosuperior iliac spine was identified. The interval between the tensor fasciae latae and the sartorius was identified and developed, taking great care not to injure the lateral femoral cutaneous nerve. The rectus femoris tendon was isolated and dissected free using blunt dissection. Two retractors were placed in the interval between the sartorius and tensor fasciae latae.

With the iliac crest held between the index finger and thumb, the iliac apophysis was incised sharply from the anterosuperior spine posteriorly to approximately the mid crest region. Then the cartilage was incised from the anterosuperior spine directly into the anteroinferior spine. Using Cobb elevators, the apophysis was "popped" off the medial and lateral aspect of the crest. Subperiosteal dissection was used to expose both the inner and outer table of the ilium. The sciatic notch was carefully exposed on the inner table of the ilium using a small Cobb elevator, taking great care not to injure the periosteum and vessels in the sciatic notch.

A quarter inch osteotome was used to outline the intended osteotomy site by cutting the cortex on the inner and outer aspect of the iliac crest. On the outer table of the ilium, the osteotomy line was curvilinear. It began about 1 cm above the anteroinferior iliac spine, passed 1.5 cm superior to the joint capsule and ended at the posterior arm of the triradiate cartilage. This was identified on fluoroscopy.

From the inner aspect, the osteotomy was carried parallel to the hip joint and then into the posterior column anterior to the notch. After the osteotomy was outlined on the inner and outer table, a wider straight osteotome was used in the anterior aspect of the osteotomy to connect the two inner and outer precut marks. As the posterior aspect of the hip joint is approached, curved osteotomes were used to continue the osteotomy into the posterior column. Special right angled osteotomes (Pemberton osteotomes) were then inserted into the osteotomy as it continued posteriorly into the posterior column. A cervical lamina spreader and cervical bone tamps of varying size were used to hold the osteotomy open while the remainder of the cuts using a Pemberton osteotome were completed into the posterior column. Fluoroscopy was used to document the location of the osteotomes and to make certain that the osteotomy was carried into the posterior aspect of the horizontal limb of the triradiate cartilage. Once the osteotomy was completed, a small groove was performed in the superior aspect of the osteotomy and a similar notch in the inferior aspect to allow for stabilization of the bone graft. A triangular wedge of bone was cut from the anterior iliac crest, grasped with a Kocher hemostat, and placed into the osteotomy gap and into the precut grooves in the superior and inferior aspects of the osteotomy site. The osteotomy was judged to be stable. The wound is then irrigated with copious amounts of saline. The iliac crest is resutured with interrupted 0 Vicryl sutures, the subcutaneous tissues with 2-0 Vicryl, and the skin closed with subcuticular 3-0 Monocryl. The wound is dressed with Steri-strips, and a Bioclusive dressing or a standard sterile dressing. The patient is then placed in a well-padded 1½ hip spica cast, extubated and taken to the postoperative recovery room.

Postoperative care: hip spica is removed in 6 weeks.

Chapter 6
Acetabular Shelf

Said Saghieh, M.D.

COMMON INDICATIONS
- Deficient acetabulum and a large femoral head with a hip that has aspherical congruity.
- Perthes Disease (Catterall Groups 2, 3, and 4; Lateral pillar B and C; Salter-Thompson B disease) in children >8 years old.

POSSIBLE COMPLICATIONS
- Pain
- Lateral femoral cutaneous nerve injury
- Infection
- Loss of range of motion
- Arthritis

ESSENTIAL STEPS
1. Bikini skin incision.
2. Split the apophysis to bone
3. Identify and avoid lateral femoral cutaneous nerve.
4. Open the sartorius and tensor fascia interval.
5. Section of the reflected head of rectus femoris.
6. Expose the capsule and identify the acetabular edge (radiographically assisted).
7. Make an up-sloping trough at the acetabular edge (drill and rongeur).
8. Obtain cortical and cancellous strips from the crest ending above the acetabular edge.
9. Cut graft to no greater than 1 cm in width and appropriate length for coverage.

S. Saghieh et al. (eds.), *Operative Dictations in Orthopedic Surgery*,
DOI 10.1007/978-1-4614-7479-1_6,
© Springer Science+Business Media New York 2013

10. Place the corticocancellous strips with cortical side down in the slot.
11. Suture the rectus tendon, holding the grafts in place.
12. Place cancellous graft on top of the corticocancellous strips.
13. Close the crest, subcutaneous layer, and skin.

OPERATIVE NOTE

Preoperative Diagnosis: Rt/Lt Perthes' disease with enlarged uncovered femoral head
Procedure: Rt/Lt; Acetabular Shelf Procedure
Postoperative Diagnosis: Same
Indications: Patient is an…year…-month-old male who has had a…month history of worsening Rt/Lt hip pain. He was found to have Perthes' disease with a mushroom deformity and lateral subluxation of the femoral head. After discussion of risks and benefits of continuing conservative treatment vs. operative procedure, the family decided to proceed with surgery.
Description of Operation: The patient was identified and the extremity marked in the preoperative holding area. He/she was brought into the operative suite and placed supine on the operating table.

General endotracheal anesthesia was induced without difficulty. IV antibiotics were administered and a Foley catheter was inserted under sterile technique.

A large bump was placed underneath patient's buttock. All bony prominences were well padded. The *Rt/Lt* flank and the entire right/left leg were prepped and draped in normal sterile fashion.

Arthrogram of the hip joint was performed under fluoroscopy. There was no evidence of hinged abduction.

A Bikini incision 2 cm below and parallel to the iliac crest was then made approximately 6 cm in length. This was carried down sharply through the subcutaneous tissue.

The cartilaginous iliac apophysis was splitted longitudinally with a scalpel. The outer half was taken down subperiosteally along the anterolateral surface of the iliac wing. The interval between the sartorius and tensor fascia interval was identified and the lateral femoral cutaneous nerve was displaced medially.

The tendon of the reflected head of rectus femoris was transected sharply and blunt dissection was utilized to separate the proximal stump from the hip capsule and reflect it posteriorly. The capsule was then exposed. It was elevated from the ilium with a periosteal elevator and reflected distally to the acetabular rim.

Under fluoroscopy, a smooth kirschner wire was introduced at the superior margin of the acetabulum. It served as a guide for drilling multiple holes of 1 cm depth with a 5/32-in. bit. A small rongeur was used to join these holes and make a slot.

Next osteotomes were utilized to harvest corticocancellous strips of the outer wall of the iliac wing. These strips were fashioned to be 1 cm in width and 1–2 mm in thickness. Cancellous bone was harvested next with curettes and gauges. A first layer of 1 mm thickness strips was inserted into the previously made trough with the cortical side lying inferiorly. Then a second layer of 2 mm thickness strips was placed above and at right angles to the first layer. The rectus stump was then pulled forward and sutured back to the rectus femoris body with 0 Vicryl. The remainder of the cortical cancellous as well as cancellous bone graft was utilized to pack the area between the iliac crest and the newly created shelf.

Fluoroscopic picture was then obtained to confirm good position of the shelf. Once this was accomplished, the wound was copiously irrigated with normal saline and then the wound was closed in three layers with fascial layer being closed with 0 Vicryl, subcutaneous layer with running 2-0 Vicryl and then the skin was closed with running subcuticular Monocryl 4-0. Wound was dressed with Steri-strips.

The kid was then placed on a hip spica table where one and a half leg spica cast was applied with the involved hip in 15° of abduction and 20° of flexion and internal rotation.

Once the cast hardens, the patient was put again on the operative table where he/she was awakened from general endotracheal anesthesia and transferred to the recovery room in excellent condition without any evidence of immediate complications.

Dr. .... was present and scrubbed for the entire procedure.

Chapter 7
Percutaneous Epiphysiodesis

Said Saghieh, M.D.

COMMON INDICATIONS
- Limb length inequality
- Infantile or adolescent Blount's disease
- Posteromedial bowing of the tibia
- Post physeal fracture

POSSIBLE COMPLICATIONS
- Continued growth of the physis
- Angular deformity
- Entering the distal femoral notch
- Fracture
- Decreased stature

ESSENTIAL STEPS
1. Position patient with a sandbag under operative side buttock.
2. Identify the level of the physis radiographically.
3. Make a small stab incision on the lateral side of the distal femur over the mid-portion of the physis in the AP dimension.
4. Introduce the guide pin then overdrill with a cannulated reamer.
5. Using the largest curette that will fit in the starting hole, scrap out the physis.
6. Once done, repeat the same steps on the proximal tibia using medial approach.
7. Make a 2 cm skin incision just proximal to the fibula head.

S. Saghieh et al. (eds.), *Operative Dictations in Orthopedic Surgery*,
DOI 10.1007/978-1-4614-7479-1_7,
© Springer Science+Business Media New York 2013

8. Introduce the guide pin across the physis followed by the reamer and the tap.
9. Insert a 4 mm cannulated partially threaded screw.
10. Close the wounds.

OPERATIVE NOTE

Preoperative Diagnosis: Limb length discrepancy of --- cm

Procedure: Combined distal femur and proximal tibia epiphysiodesis, r/l.

Postoperative Diagnosis: Same

Indications: Patient is a ....-year-old male/female who has a -- cm limb length discrepancy. According to the preoperative planning, combined distal femur and proximal tibia epiphysiodesis at this age, would allow the patient to have equal legs length at maturity.

Description of Operation: Patient was identified as the correct person in the preoperative holding area and brought into the operative suite and placed supine on the operating table where he/she was induced into general endotracheal anesthesia. All bony prominences well padded. No tourniquet was used. The patient was given IV Antibiotics.

Patient's *Rt/Lt* leg was then prepped and draped in the normal sterile fashion. Fluoroscopic guidance was utilized to identify the level of the growth plate of the distal femur. A stab wound was performed on the lateral side of the growth plate and deepened through subcutaneous tissue and the fascia lata down to the level of the bone. A smooth guide pin was placed under fluoroscopic control as central as it can be in the growth plate. It was over-drilled with a 8 mm cannulated reamer. The pin was removed and the tunnel was further widened using adequate curve curette. The curettage confirmed the presence of cartilage of the physis. After irrigation, the wound was closed in one layer with staples.

Then the physis of the proximal tibia was identified with the use of fluoroscopy. A stab wound was performed on its medial side. Blunt dissection was carried through the subcutaneous tissues down to the level of the bone. A guide pin was introduced and its central position verified with fluoroscopy to be central. The 8 mm cannulated reamer was used again to drill over the guide pin. Curettes were used in a similar manner. The wound was closed with two staples.

Finally, a 2 cm longitudinal skin incision was made at the level of the fibula head. A guide wire was introduced through the head and across the physis into the intramedullary canal of the fibula. A 3.2 mm cannulated reamer was used to drill over the guide wire.

The tunnel was tapped and a 30 mm 4.0 mm cannulated partially threaded screw was used to compress the physis.

The wound was irrigated and closed in two layers; the subcutaneous tissue with vicryl 3.0 and the skin with 4-0 monocryl. The wounds were dressed with steri-strips, xeroform and kerlex. The patient was placed into a soft bulky Jones dressing, awakened from general anesthesia and taken to the recovery room in excellent condition without evidence of immediate complications.

Dr. .... was present and scrubbed for the entire procedure.

Chapter 8
Proximal Femoral Osteotomy

Joseph G. Khoury, M.D.

COMMON INDICATIONS
- Developmental dysplasia of the hip, Perthes disease, congenital coxa vara, segmental AVN, and more

Of note: there are many different types and locations of osteotomies at the proximal femur. We will describe the varus osteotomy done for DDH

POSSIBLE COMPLICATIONS
- Altered lever arm for the abductors
- Altered knee joint alignment
- AVN

ESSENTIAL STEPS
1. Incision from tip of greater trochanter down in line with the shaft
2. Divide fascia lata in line with incision
3. Detach vastus lateralis from vastus ridge and retract anterior
4. Judge anteversion with k-wire along anterior neck
5. Determine angle of blade insertion based on pre-op planning
6. Insert blade into the head at correct angle
7. Make cut at preplanned level (usually just above lesser troch)
8. Bring down the blade and secure to the shaft, derotate as needed
9. Check position with fluoro

S. Saghieh et al. (eds.), *Operative Dictations in Orthopedic Surgery*,
DOI 10.1007/978-1-4614-7479-1_8,
© Springer Science+Business Media New York 2013

OPERATIVE NOTE

Preoperative Diagnosis: Developmental dysplasia of the hip with subluxation

Procedure: Varus osteotomy of the proximal femur

Postoperative Diagnosis: Same

Indications: This 4-year-old child diagnosed with DDH at birth has undergone closed reduction at 3 months of age. Her acetabulum has failed to develop adequately and her hip is slightly subluxated. Abduction views showed that the head can be well contained. Her neck shaft angle appears to be 150°. After discussion with her parents, the decision was made to proceed with varus osteotomy of the proximal femur to redirect the femoral head deep into the acetabulum.

Description of Operation: The patient was properly identified by anesthesia and positioned supine on the flat table. Anesthesia was administered. The hip was bumped and prepped/draped in the usual fashion. A longitudinal incision was made from the tip of the greater trochanter, 8 in. along the shaft. The fascia lata was divided in line with the incision. The vastus lateralis was detached from its origin at the vastus ridge and retracted anteriorly with a homan retractor placed directly on the anterior femur. The anterior neck was bluntly dissected and with a finger along the neck, a k-wire was directed along the anterior neck into the head. A guide wire was inserted into the tip of the greater trochanter and a second wire near the knee to subtend the intended arc of derotation. A guide wire for the cannulated blade plate was inserted up the femoral neck from superolateral (just below the lateral edge of the greater trochanteric apophysis) to inferomedial at a 20° angle against the axis of the femoral neck (for a final neck shaft angle of 110°). The position of the wire in the center of the next was confirmed on frog lateral fluoroscopy. Next, the chisel was inserted over the wire 10 mm at a time and removed in order to prevent incarceration of the chisel. With retractors around the femur, the cut was made 1 cm below the blade insertion site. The blade was then inserted over the wire. The neck was tipped into varus until the plate came into contact with the distal fragment with the femoral shaft slightly displaced medially. The distal fragment was rotated until the reference wires are parallel. The plate was secured with screws. Final position was confirmed with fluoroscopy. The wound was irrigated with sterile saline. The vastus was re-approximated with 0-vicryl interrupted sutures. The fascia lata was closed with a running 0-vicryl and the subcutaneus layer with a running 2-0 vicryl. The skin was closed with a running 3-0 monocryl subcuticular stitch and steri-strips. A sterile dressing was applied and then a one and one-half hip spica cast.

Chapter 9
Hamstring Lengthening

Said Saghieh, M.D.

COMMON INDICATIONS

- Cerebral palsy patient. Hamstrings lengthening can be isolated or combined with other tendons lengthening.
- Extreme contractures of the knee that impair sitting may be indicated for hamstring lengthening even in a non-ambulatory patients.

POSSIBLE COMPLICATIONS

- Recurvatum at the knee if the hamstrings are overly weakened and/or the quadriceps are severely spastic.
- Direct injury to the peroneal nerve when manipulating the biceps femoris.
- Indirect injury to the popliteal artery or sciatic nerve from the correction (i.e., stretch injury).

ESSENTIAL STEPS

1. Prone positioning in isolated hamstring lengthening.
2. A single midline longitudinal incision just superior to the popliteal fossa.
3. Identification of the three hamstrings.
4. Z-plasty of the semitendinosis.
5. Fractional lengthening of the semimembranosis and the biceps femoris.
6. Apply cast in amount of extension that can be obtained without force.

S. Saghieh et al. (eds.), *Operative Dictations in Orthopedic Surgery*,
DOI 10.1007/978-1-4614-7479-1_9,
© Springer Science+Business Media New York 2013

OPERATIVE NOTE

Preoperative Diagnosis: Cerebral palsy patient who walks with a thirty degree bent knee. No flexion contracture of the hip. No equinus deformity

Procedure: Hamstrings lengthening

Postoperative Diagnosis: Same

Description of Operation: The patient was brought to the operating room supine on the stretcher. IV antibiotics were given, and a well-padded thigh tourniquet was placed. After adequate general anesthesia was provided, the patient was rolled to the prone position on the operative table and all pressure points were padded.

The patient lower extremity was then prepped and draped in the standard surgical fashion.

The lower extremity was exsanguinated with an Esmarch bandage and the tourniquet was inflated to 300 mm Hg. A 10 cm midline, longitudinal skin incision was performed starting proximal to the polpliteal crease. The subcutaneous fat was divided protecting the posterior femoral cutaneous nerve in the proximal portion of the wound. The semitendinosis was identified medially. A Z-lengthening of the tendon was performed. The semimembranosis was then identified deep to the semitendinosis. A fractional lengthening was performed at the musculotendinous junction with the tendinous portion divided transversely at two levels, 3 cm apart.

The biceps femoris was then identified on the lateral side. A similar fractional lengthening was done taking into consideration to stay away from the common peroneal nerve.

The wound was then irrigated. The tourniquet was deflated and hemostasis obtained with electrocautery. The subcutaneous tissue was closed with 2.0 vicryl placed in a simple fashion. The skin was closed with 4-0 monocryl in subcuticular fashion. A clean dressing was applied, followed by a long leg cylinder cast.

The patient was extubated and taken to the postoperative recovery room in good conditions.

No intraoperative complications.

Staff was present and scrubbed for entire procedure.

AFTER TREATMENT

The patient is allowed to walk with crutches with weight bearing as tolerated. The cast is removed in 4 weeks and physical therapy started.

Knee immobilizers are used for approximately 8–12 weeks postoperatively.

Chapter 10
Tibia Spike Osteotomy for Genu Varum

Said Saghieh, M.D.

COMMON INDICATIONS
- Genu varum of different etiologies including Blount's disease.
- The same osteotomy can be performed for other angular deformities of long bones with reversal of the spike location.
- Age: preferably done in skeletally immature patients.

POSSIBLE COMPLICATIONS
- Wound infection, osteomyelitis.
- Nerve injury, compartment syndrome.
- Fractures.
- Secondary displacement.
- Recurrence of the deformity in growing kids.

ESSENTIAL STEPS
1. Preoperative planning.
2. Supine position on a radiolucent table.
3. Fibula osteotomy.
4. Incision on the medial side of the proximal tibia.
5. Outline the osteotomy with drill holes
6. Completion of the osteotomy.
7. Angular correction.
8. Cast application.

S. Saghieh et al. (eds.), *Operative Dictations in Orthopedic Surgery*,
DOI 10.1007/978-1-4614-7479-1_10,
© Springer Science+Business Media New York 2013

OPERATIVE NOTE

Preoperative Diagnosis: Tibia Vara
Procedure: Tibia spike osteotomy
Postoperative Diagnosis: Tibia vara
Description of Operation: The patient was brought to the operating room and placed supine on the operating table. After adequate general anesthesia was provided, a well-padded thigh tourniquet was placed. The lower extremity was then prepped and draped in the standard surgical fashion.

The lower extremity was exsanguinated with an Esmarch bandage and the tourniquet was inflated to 250 mm Hg. A 15 blade was used to make a 5 cm longitudinal incision in the middle third of the leg over the fibula. The bone was exposed subperiosteally and a 2 cm segment was resected. Prophylactic anterior compartment fasciotomy was next performed. The wound was closed in two layers: vicryl 3.0 for the subcutaneous tissue and monocryl 4.0 for the skin.

Then an 8 cm medial, longitudinal incision centered on the metaphyseal diaphyseal junction of the proximal tibia was made. A circumferential periosteal stripping of the bone was performed.

The osteotomy was outlined with 2.5 mm anteroposterior drill holes. The holes started medially, crossed the midline perpendicular to the axis of the bone before shaping the spike on the lateral side. The spike had a height of (3–4) cm and a base of (1–1.5) cm. The drill holes were connected with an osteotome taking care not to fracture the spike. Once the osteotomy was completed, the distal fragment was angulated laterally and the spike was impaled into the cancellous bone of the metaphysis. Fluoroscopy confirmed the adequacy of the correction.

The wound was thoroughly irrigated with saline and was closed in anatomic layers; the periosteum with interrupted 2.0 vicryl, the subcutaneous tissue with 3.0 vicryl and the skin with monocryl 4.0.

A long leg cast was applied to maintain the correction. Fluoroscopy was used again to assess the fragments position before extubation of the patient.

Dr. .... was present and scrubbed for the entire procedure.

Chapter 11
Closed Manipulation and Tenotomy for Clubfoot

Mark L. Hagy, M.D.

COMMON INDICATIONS
- Correction of clubfoot foot deformity

POSSIBLE COMPLICATIONS
- Skin breakdown
- Failure of correction
- Recurrence

ESSENTIAL STEPS
1. First cast in supination
2. Series of 3–4 abduction casts changed at weekly interval
3. Percutaneous Achilles tenotomy to correct equinus
4. Denis-Browne splint

OPERATIVE NOTE
Preoperative Diagnosis: Clubfoot
Procedure: Ponseti method for correction of clubfoot
Postoperative Diagnosis: Same
Description of Operation:
   First cast: Start as soon after birth as possible. The child is brought to the procedure room. No anesthetic needed. Allow the infant to feed during the casting process.

   The first metatarsal is elevated and the forefoot is supinated to realign the forefoot with the hindfoot and correct the cavus.

   Soft roll is applied from the tip of the toes to the proximal thigh. Care is taken to avoid excessive padding. Plaster is applied

S. Saghieh et al. (eds.), *Operative Dictations in Orthopedic Surgery*,
DOI 10.1007/978-1-4614-7479-1_11,
© Springer Science+Business Media New York 2013

as a below-knee cast. After the plaster sets, the cast is extended to the upper third of the thigh with the knee flexed to 90° and the tibia slightly externally rotated. Anatomic molding is carried out in the popliteal fossa.

The child is kept in the waiting area for 15 min to make sure that the cast is not too tight before discharging him/her home.

Second to fourth cast: The child is brought to the procedure room. No anesthetic needed. Allow the infant to feed during the manipulation and casting processes.

The talar head is localized in front of the lateral malleolus. It is stabilized by the thumb while the index of the same hand is placed behind the lateral malleolus. The foot is then abducted as far as can be done without causing discomfort to the infant. The pressure is maintained for 1 min. After 3–4 manipulations, soft roll is applied from the tip of the toes to the proximal thigh. Care is taken to avoid excessive padding. Plaster is applied as a below-knee cast while the foot is abducted and counterpressure is applied over the head of the talus serving as a fulcrum. The cast is molded gently along the Achilles tendon and the malleoli. After the plaster sets, the cast is extended to the upper third of the thigh with the knee flexed to 90° and the tibia slightly externally rotated. Anatomic molding is carried out in the popliteal fossa.

The child is kept in the waiting area for 15 min to make sure that the cast is not too tight before discharging him/her home.

Similarly, the child returns on a weekly basis for removal of the cast and progressive correction with further abduction. Once the foot reaches 70° of external rotation, usually after 3–4 casts, tenotomy is done.

Achilles tenotomy: Emla gel is applied over the posterior ankle for 15 min. Then the child is placed prone and the foot (or feet) is prepped and draped in a sterile fashion. A beaver blade (size) is introduced medial to the Achilles tendon, 1.5 cm above the calcaneus. Once it reaches its deeper surface, it is turned 90° and used to perform complete tenotomy while dorsiflexion force is applied to the ankle. The knife is withdrawn, pressure is applied to the wound for 5 min to stop the bleeding, a steristrip adhesive is applied.

A long leg cast is applied with the ankle abducted 60–70° and dorsiflexed 10–15° and the knee flexed 90°.

Postoperative care: The last cast applied for 3 weeks.

Following casting the child remains in a Denis-Browne Bar with the involved foot in 60–70° of external rotation for 3 months at all times, followed by use at night and naptime over the next 2–3 years in order to prevent recurrence.

Chapter 12
Posteromedial Release for Clubfoot

Joseph G. Khoury, M.D.

COMMON INDICATIONS
- Failed casting
- Older child at presentation
- Teratologic clubfoot

POSSIBLE COMPLICATIONS
- Skin slough
- Injury to medial neurovascular structures
- Instability from release of too much deltoid ligament
- Dividing the cartilagenous neck of the talus

ESSENTIAL STEPS
1. There are numerous incisions described and this is a topic of great debate.
2. The remaining steps are done in sequence as needed. Not all may be needed.

POSTERIOR RELEASE
1. Expose achilles tendon within the sheath
2. Z-lengthening of the achilles tendon. Repair later
3. Open posterior compartment (looking for FHL)
4. Subperiosteal dissection under FHL around medial side of ankle and subtalar joint
5. Open peroneal tendon sheath to tip of lateral malleolus
6. Release underneath up to and including the calcaneofibular ligament
7. Incise the capsule in the entire area just exposed

S. Saghieh et al. (eds.), *Operative Dictations in Orthopedic Surgery,*
DOI 10.1007/978-1-4614-7479-1_12,

MEDIAL RELEASE

1. Release proximal attachment of abductor hallucis
2. Expose FDL and tibialis posterior from the medial malleolus to the knot of Henry
3. Detach posterior tibial tendon
4. Open the talonavicular joint capsule including spring ligament and anterior fibers of deltoid
5. Open the calcaneocuboid joint capsule
6. Divide plantar fascia behind the neurovascular bundle, just off the insertion of the calcaneus
7. Pin talonavicular joint
8. Second pin from calcaneus, through talus, into the tibia
9. Reattach PTT. Lengthen FHL and FDL together

LATERAL RELEASE

1. Shorten lateral column either through either the calcaneocuboid joint or bone.

OPERATIVE NOTE

Preoperative Diagnosis: Clubfoot
Procedure: Posteromedial release of clubfoot
Postoperative Diagnosis: Same
Indications: This 10-month-old child has failed multiple attempts at treatment with manipulation and long leg casting. This foot is very stiff and resistant to treatment. After discussion with his parents, the decision was made to proceed with surgical correction.
Description of Operation: The patient is positioned prone. The leg was elevated and exsanguinated with the use of an Esmarch and tourniquet inflated to 220 mmHg. A posteromedial incision was made. Dissection was carried down through subcutaneous tissues and the neurovascular bundle was identified and dissected along its course and gently retracted with a vessel loop. The posterior tibial, FDL, and FHL tendons were identified and retracted. The tendon Achilles was then identified. The sheath was opened and the achilles tendon was subsequently divided in a Z-lengthening fashion. The posterior ankle capsule was identified and cleared of both posteromedial and posterolateral structures. The neurovascular bundle and tendons were protected while the capsule was incised into the tibiotalar and subtalar joints. Care was taken to protect the cartilagenous surfaces at this point. Next, the PTT was taken off the navicular taking care to protect the insertion of peroneus longus. The FDL and FHL were traced from the malleolus to the knot of Henry and sewn together on the plantar aspect of the

foot. These were then divided in a z-fashion for later repair. The plantar fascia was release just off the calcaneus behind the neurovascular bundle with a retractor protecting it. The talonavicular and calcaneocuboid joint capsules were opened completely. The foot was noted to be plantigrade at this point in time and the wound was then thoroughly irrigated. We did not feel a lateral column shortening would be needed. A 0.062 K-wire was passed up the calcaneus and the tibia, holding the foot in appropriate position. A second wire held the talonavicular joint in a reduced position. The wound was then closed with 2-0 Vicryl approximating the subcutaneous fat and 4-0 Monocryl approximating the skin edges in a subcuticular manner. The wound was then cleaned and covered with sterile bandages. The leg was then overwrapped with Xeroform and sterile Sof-Rol and a short leg cast was then applied. The patient was then taken to the recovery room where recovery was uneventful, and subsequently was admitted to the floor for postoperative care.

Chapter 13

Anterior Tibialis Transfer to the Lateral Cuneiform

Said Saghieh, M.D.

COMMON INDICATIONS
- Dynamic supination after correction of clubfoot deformity
- Muscle imbalance

POSSIBLE COMPLICATIONS
- Residual or recurrent deformity
- Weakness of dorsiflexion
- Persistent muscle imbalance
- Tendon pull out

ESSENTIAL STEPS
1. Position patient supine.
2. Incise longitudinally along medial border of the anterior tibial tendon.
3. Dissect out the tendon as distal as possible before disinsertion.
4. Incise longitudinally over the third cuneiform.
5. Drill a hole in a dorsal to plantar direction through the cuneiform with a 3/8″ drill bit.
6. Pass the tendon from medial to lateral deep to the extensor retinaculum.
7. Pass the suture through the bone hole out to the plantar aspect of the foot.
8. Feed the tendon into the bone hole as the suture is pulled taught.

S. Saghieh et al. (eds.), *Operative Dictations in Orthopedic Surgery*,
DOI 10.1007/978-1-4614-7479-1_13,
© Springer Science+Business Media New York 2013

9. Tie the suture over adaptic, sterile foam, and then a button.
10. Hold the foot dorsiflexed again while irrigating and closing the incision.
11. Apply long leg cast in slight dorsiflexion.

OPERATIVE NOTE

Preoperative Diagnosis: Dynamic supination of the—foot
Procedure: Anterior tibialis tendon transfer to the third cuneiform
Postoperative Diagnosis: Same
Indications: Patient is a ---- old b/g who was treated for l/r clubfoot deformity and who developed dynamic supination of the foot. We discussed with the parents the benefit of anterior tibialis tendon transfer.
Description of Operation: The patient was identified and the extremity marked in the preoperative holding area. He/she was brought into the operative suite and placed supine on the operating table. The patient was induced into general endotracheal anesthesia without difficulty. IV antibiotics were administered. All bony prominences of the patient were well padded and protected. A tourniquet was placed on the patient's left/right proximal thigh over soft roll, and the extremity was prepped and draped in the normal sterile fashion.

The tourniquet was placed up to 220 mm of mercury.

A 5 cm longitudinal skin incision was made medial and parallel to the distal part of the tibialis anterior, and sharp dissection was carried down to the level of the tendon sheath. The tendon sheath was incised longitudinally, and the tibialis anterior tendon was isolated. The tibialis anterior tendon was dissected off its insertion as distally as possible. Two Keith needles were used to place a stay stitch on the tendon.

Next, a longitudinal incision was made over the third cuneiform. The extensor tendons were mobilized and the third cuneiform was identified with fluoroscopy. Sharp dissection was carried down to the level of the periosteum. A periosteal elevator was utilized to move any periosteum and cartilage that was overlying the bone. A 3/8″ hand drill was then utilized to make a hole in the third cuneiform from dorsal to plantar.

Next, a hemostat was placed underneath the extensor retinaculum of the ankle proximally and spread underneath the retinaculum. The tibialis anterior tendon was grasped by the stay sutures and pulled underneath the extensor retinaculum. The two

Keith needles were replaced back onto the free ends of the sutured tibialis anterior tendon, and passed through the bony tunnel into the plantar surface of the foot and tied over adaptic sterile gauze and a button while the foot is in maximum dorsiflexion.

Both wounds were irrigated copiously with normal saline. The extensor retinaculum was closed with Vicryl 2-0, the subcutaneous with Vicryl 3-0, and the skin with 4-0 Monocryl in a running simple fashion. A sterile dressing was applied followed by a long leg cast. The tourniquet was let down. The patient was extubated and was transferred to the postoperative recovery room without any evidence of immediate complications.

Dr. .... was present and scrubbed for the entire procedure.

Chapter 14
Split Posterior Tibial Tendon Transfer

Rola H. Rashid, M.D.

COMMON INDICATIONS
- Dynamic varus deformity of the hindfoot and midfoot

POSSIBLE COMPLICATIONS
- Wound infection
- Dehiscence
- Failed transfer
- Recurrence of the deformity

ESSENTIAL STEPS
1. Posteromedial incision
2. Splitting of the posterior tibial tendon
3. Lateral incision
4. Identification of the peroneus brevis
5. Transfer of the split half of the tendon laterally to be sutured to the peroneus brevis tendon

OPERATIVE NOTE
Preoperative Diagnosis: Cerebral palsy with dynamic varus deformity

Procedure: Split posterior tibial tendon transfer

Postoperative Diagnosis: Same

Description of Operation: The patient was identified and the surgical site was marked prior to the transfer to the operating room. General anesthesia was induced by the anesthesia team.

S. Saghieh et al. (eds.), *Operative Dictations in Orthopedic Surgery*, DOI 10.1007/978-1-4614-7479-1_14,

The patient was positioned supine on the operating table. A tourniquet was applied.

IV antibiotics were administered. The extremity was prepped and draped from the knee to the toes in the usual sterile fashion.

Tourniquet was inflated to 300 mmHg.

With a 15 blade, a posteromedial ankle incision was performed. It started 7 cm proximal to the tip of the medial malleolus slightly posterior to the medial tibia cortex to terminate distally 1.5 cm below to the tip of the medial malleolus where it curved anteriorly to terminate 1 cm distal to the tuberosity of the navicular.

The posterior tibial tendon was identified behind the posteromedial margin of the tibia. The sheath was incised. The tendon was split longitudinally into two halves by blunt dissection. The plantar half of the tendon was sectioned at its navicular insertion and pulled proximally.

A separate curvilinear lateral incision was performed. It started 3 cm proximal to the tip of the lateral malleolus slightly posterior to the fibula and curved anteriorly below the tip of the lateral malleolus to finish at the base of the fifth metatarsal.

The peroneal tendons were exposed. The sheath of the peroneus brevis was incised.

With an Ober tendon passer, the split segment of the posterior tibial tendon was passed from the medial to the lateral wound behind the tibia. It was sutured to the peroneus brevis tendon with 0 Ticron under tension.

The tourniquet was released, hemostasis was achieved, and the wound was closed in anatomical layers: subcutaneous tissue with 3-0 vicryl and skin with 4-0 monocryl.

Sterile dressings were applied followed by a short leg cast with the ankle in neutral position and the heel in slight eversion.

No intraoperative complications.

Staff was present and scrubbed for entire procedure.

Post-op regimen: cast for 3–4 weeks.

Chapter 15
In Situ Pinning of SCFE

John-Erik Bell, M.D., M.S.

COMMON INDICATIONS
- Mild to moderate SCFE
- Most authors also recommend it for severe SCFE

POSSIBLE COMPLICATIONS
- AVN
- Malunion
- Infection
- Growth arrest
- Chondrolysis
- Fracture
- Nonunion
- Hardware breakage

ESSENTIAL STEPS
1. Position—supine on fracture table—opposite leg extended and abducted.
2. Do not perform a reduction or use significant traction.
3. Check views (AP/lat) with fluoroscopy before prepping and draping. Make sure subchondral bone and physeal plate are visible.
4. Angle pin anterior to posterior.
5. Advance pin (no closer to subchondral bone than 5 mm).
6. Drill, tap, and advance screw (should be at least 6.5 mm).
7. Check screw in multiple fluoro positions to look for joint penetration.

S. Saghieh et al. (eds.), *Operative Dictations in Orthopedic Surgery*,
DOI 10.1007/978-1-4614-7479-1_15,
© Springer Science+Business Media New York 2013

OPERATIVE NOTE
Preoperative Diagnosis: SCFE
Procedure: In situ pinning of capital femoral epiphysis
Postoperative Diagnosis: Same
Description of Operation: The patient was identified and the site of surgery confirmed. Anesthesia was induced. Prophylactic antibiotics were administered. The patient was placed supine on the fracture table in minimal skin traction. The opposite leg was abducted and extended. Fluoroscopy was used to verify appropriate visualization of the hip, subchondral bone, and physeal plate in the AP and lateral planes. The patient was then prepped and draped.

A free pin was placed over the hip to verify AP orientation of the femoral neck and a line drawn along the pin. A second line was then drawn in line with the femoral neck on the lateral view. The incision was then made centered on the intersection of the lines. The incision was carried through subcutaneous tissues, the fascia, and through the vastus lateralis. Then a guide pin was inserted centered in both the AP and lateral planes, taking care to aim slightly anterior to posterior to take into account the posterior displacement of the epiphysis. The guide wire was advanced just short of the subchondral bone, measured, overdrilled, and then overtapped. A 6.5 cannulated screw was then inserted and checked fluoroscopically in multiple planes to ensure no penetration into the joint. The wound was then irrigated, closed in layers, and sterilely dressed.

Chapter 16
Closed Reduction and Percutaneous Pinning of Supracondylar Humerus Fracture

Said Saghieh, M.D.

COMMON INDICATIONS
- Type 2,3 supracondylar humerus fracture

POSSIBLE COMPLICATIONS
- Brachial artery injury
- Ulna nerve injury
- Compartment syndrome
- Secondary displacement
- Late cubitus varus

ESSENTIAL STEPS
1. Careful preoperative assessment (history, physical examination–evaluation of compartment syndrome, radiographs)
2. Closed reduction
3. Cross pinning
4. Long arm splint

OPERATIVE NOTE
Preoperative Diagnosis: Supracondylar humerus fracture (extension type)
Procedure: Closed reduction and percutaneous pinning
Postoperative Diagnosis: Same

S. Saghieh et al. (eds.), *Operative Dictations in Orthopedic Surgery*,
DOI 10.1007/978-1-4614-7479-1_16,
© Springer Science+Business Media New York 2013

Indications: ___ yo child who fell on the outstretched hand with the elbow hyperextended and sustained an extension type fracture of the supracondylar area of the distal humerus.

Description of Operation: The patient underwent anesthesia per the anesthesia team. The patient was positioned supine with the shoulder at the edge of the table and the involved extremity resting on the tube of the image intensifier. The upper extremity was prepped and draped in the usual sterile fashion.

With the elbow extended, gentle longitudinal traction was applied to the supinated forearm, with counter traction applied to the upper part of the arm by my assistant. The frontal plane displacement and the rotation were corrected while maintaining the longitudinal traction. The elbow was flexed to 120° and the forearm pronated. Fluoroscopy confirmed the reduction on the lateral view and Jones view.

The fracture was then fixed with two crossed smooth 0.062-in. K-wires. The lateral one was first inserted from the lateral epicondyle and directed cephalad and medially. Then the elbow was extended to 80°, the ulna nerve was palpated in its groove and pushed posteriorly while the medial K-wire was introduced through the medial epicondyle and directed cephalad and laterally. Fluoroscopy confirmed fracture reduction and satisfactory wires configuration.

A posterior splint was applied with the elbow flexed 90° and the forearm in neutral position. The distal pulses were palpable at the end of the procedure.

No intraoperative complications.

Staff was present and scrubbed for entire procedure.

Post-op regimen: Hospitalization 24–48 h with strict elevation of the upper extremity. The patient needs K-wires removal under general anesthesia in 3 weeks.

Chapter 17

Open Reduction and Internal Fixation of Supracondylar Humerus Fracture

Said Saghieh, M.D.

COMMON INDICATIONS
- Type 3 supracondylar humerus fracture

POSSIBLE COMPLICATIONS
- Brachial artery injury
- Ulna nerve injury
- Compartment syndrome
- Infection
- Secondary displacement
- Late cubitus varus

ESSENTIAL STEPS
1. Careful preoperative assessment (history, physical examination–evaluation of neurovascular structures, radiographs)
2. Attempt for closed reduction
3. Open reduction through medial, possible lateral incision
4. Cross pinning
5. Long arm splint

OPERATIVE NOTE
Preoperative Diagnosis: Supracondylar humerus fracture (extension type 3)
Procedure: Open reduction and internal fixation

S. Saghieh et al. (eds.), *Operative Dictations in Orthopedic Surgery*,
DOI 10.1007/978-1-4614-7479-1_17,
© Springer Science+Business Media New York 2013

Postoperative Diagnosis: Same

Indications: ___ yo child who fell on the outstretched hand with the elbow hyperextended and sustained an extension type 3 fracture of the supracondylar area of the distal humerus.

Description of Operation: The patient underwent general anesthesia per the anesthesia team. The patient was positioned supine with the shoulder at the edge of the table and the involved extremity resting on a radiolucent arm table. The upper extremity was prepped and draped in the usual sterile fashion.

Under fluoroscopy control, closed reduction of the fracture was attempted unsuccessfully.

A longitudinal incision 3- to 4-cm long was made over the medial side of the distal end of the humerus and elbow. The subcutaneous fat was incised, the ulna nerve pushed posteriorly and the fracture identified. There was no neural or vascular structure entrapped between the two fragments. The fracture was then reduced and fixed with one smooth 0.062-in. K-wire. Fluoroscopy control showed significant residual rotation of the distal fragment.

A lateral longitudinal incision was made over the lateral condyle of the distal end of the humerus to allow exposure of the lateral side of the fracture. Reduction was achieved successfully under direct vision from both wounds. The medial K-wire was repositioned and a similar lateral one was inserted from the lateral epicondyle and oriented medially and cephalad.

Fluoroscopy confirmed fracture reduction and satisfactory wires configuration. The two wires crossed proximal to the fracture side.

The wires were bent and buried under the skin. The incisions were closed in two layers; the subcutaneous layer with 3-0 vicryl and the skin with 4-0 monocryl in subcuticular fashion.

The wounds were covered with steri-strip s and a sterile dressing. A posterior splint was applied with the elbow in 90° of flexion and the forearm in neutral position.

The distal pulses were palpable at the end of the procedure.

No intraoperative complications.

Staff was present and scrubbed for entire procedure.

Post-op regimen: Hospitalization 24–48 h with strict elevation of the upper extremity. The patient needs K-wires removal under general anesthesia in 3 weeks.

Part II
Spine

Chapter 18
Laminotomy and Partial Discectomy for Lumbar Disc Herniation

Anthony V. Mollano, M.D.

COMMON INDICATIONS
- Positive myelogram/MRI correlating with clinical findings
- Weakness consistent with positive EMG
- Positive crossed straight-leg-raise sign
- Failure to respond to a minimum of 1 month of nonoperative management
- Impaired quality of life
- Absence of personality and thought disorders
- Absence of an engaged attorney

POSSIBLE COMPLICATIONS
- Recurrent disc herniation
- Nerve root injury
- Peri-neural scar formation
- Lateral femoral cutaneous nerve paresthesia
- Dural tear
- Brachial plexus traction injury
- Epidural hematoma
- Wound infection
- Epidural abscess
- Meningitis
- Vertebral osteomyelitis
- Major vessel injury or visceral injury with concomitant high mortality risk
- Cauda equina syndrome (from epidural hematoma or injured artery of Adamkiewicz).

S. Saghieh et al. (eds.), *Operative Dictations in Orthopedic Surgery*,
DOI 10.1007/978-1-4614-7479-1_18,
© Springer Science+Business Media New York 2013

ESSENTIAL STEPS

1. Administer general anesthesia.
2. Place patient prone on a Wilson frame in slight hip flexion, check positioning and all pressure points, and sterilely prep and drape.
3. Palpate iliac crests, and mark target level with pen.
4. Make vertical midline incision over spinous processes, and then dissect lateral to spinous processes on affected side down to laminae using electrocautery, and a Cobb elevator for retraction.
5. Place towel clip at target level, and obtain lateral radiograph for level confirmation.
6. For patient with L4/L5 disc herniation causing L5 radiculopathy, examine interlaminar space, and perform partial laminotomy involving the caudal 3 mm of L4 and the cranial 3 mm of L5, if necessary.
7. Strip ligamentum flavum with Penfield 1 elevator from respective laminae above and below target disc.
8. For exposure, remove additional respective portions of laminae and medial facet joint capsule, with upbiting rongeur, if necessary, then expose dura, and dissect from medial portion of dura laterally to identify the affected nerve root (with care to not mistake the lateral border of the dura for the nerve root when disc herniations occur medial to the nerve root).
9. For disc extrusions (75 % of lumbar herniations) remove visible disc material, and for disc protrusions, perform sharp cruciate annulotomy with subsequent partial discectomy.
10. Inspect neural foramina, check that nerve root remains free from tension allowing for at least 1 cm of medial displacement, irrigate wound, and place fat graft.
11. Close in layers with figure-8 sutures for watertight fascia seal, close skin with subcutaneous stitches, apply sterile bandage, roll and transfer patient to bed, and extubate.

OPERATIVE NOTE

Preoperative Diagnosis: L4/L5 disc herniation with L5 radiculopathy

Procedure: L4/L5 laminotomy and partial discectomy

Postoperative Diagnosis: Same

Indications: A healthy X-year-old patient with buttock pain radiating down to the great toe. Pain exacerbating with coughing and straining. Onset was acute 2 months ago with lifting heavy box. Quality of life impaired with inability to work desk job. Conservative therapy unsuccessful. MRI demonstrates large posterolateral L4/L5 disc herniation impinging on L5 nerve root. The patient understood the risks and benefits of surgery and elected to proceed.

Description of Operation: General anesthesia was administered with the patient supine, with endotracheal intubation without difficulty. The patient was gently log-rolled to and positioned prone on the Wilson frame. Care was taken to protect and pad all pressure points. The back was sterilely prepped and draped. A midline longitudinal incision was made over the lumbosacral junction. Sharp dissection was carried through subcutaneous tissue with hemostasis controlled with electrocoagulation. Supraspinous ligament and thoracodorsal fascia were identified and incised in the midline. Paraspinal muscles were subperiosteally elevated from the (affected) lateral side of the spinous processes at that level. A lateral radiograph was taken to assist with level identification between the spinous processes of L4 and L5. The undersurface of the caudal portion of the lamina of L4 and the cranial 3 mm of L5 were cleared. A laminotomy involving the caudal 3 mm of L4 and the cranial 3 mm of L5 were then undertaken. The borders of the ligamentum flavum were then identified and separated from the lamina. Ligamentum flavum was detached from its insertion into the medial facet capsule and reflected toward the midline. Portions of the medial facet capsule were removed to allow satisfactory visualization laterally. Upon entrance to the epidural space, the contents of the canal were protected at all times with square cottonoid patties. The thecal sac was then identified and its lateral border was gently teased free. It was retracted toward the midline and there was immediate visualization of a large extruded disc portion within the canal. The L5 nerve root was identified and retracted toward the midline. Large epidural bleeders were controlled with bipolar electrocoagulation. With gentle retraction toward the midline, the thecal sac and root were retracted toward the midline with a D'Errico nerve root retractor. A cruciate incision was made in fibrinous material overlying the disc material and there was immediate expression of disc material through the cruciate incision. Multiple fragments of disc material were removed including the largest ones measuring approximately .... After removal of the disc material within the canal, the floor of the canal was inspected and found to be quite flattened. The opposing layers of fibrinous outer annulus were laying flat. The posterior boundary of the body of L5 and S1 were probed and found to be free. A Murphy ball-tip probe could then be easily passed in all four quadrants about the nerve root. It could easily pass ventral to the thecal sac. The wound was irrigated with antibiotic irrigant. The patient underwent forceful Valsava maneuver and there was no expression of CSF. A fat graft was harvested subcutaneously. The exposed thecal sac and root were bathed with combined depo-medrol and marcaine. The ligamentum flavum flap was then allowed to fall back onto the dura. Exposed boundaries of the thecal sac were covered with subcutaneous fat graft. The Taylor retractor was removed and the paraspinal muscles allowed to fall into their anatomic position. The supraspinous ligament was reapproximated with multiple 0-Vicryl figure-of-eight sutures. Subcutaneous tissue was closed in layers with 2-0 Vicryl followed by a 3-0 Monocryl running suture for skin closure. Steri-strips and sterile dressings were applied. The patient was gently log-rolled, transferred to a hospital bed, extubated, positioned with the head of bed elevated, and transferred to the recovery room in stable condition. Sponge and needle counts were correct, times two. Loupe magnification and high intensity illumination were employed at all times. Specimen of the L4/L5 disc material was sent for gross pathology only.

Dr. Staff Faculty Surgeon was present, scrubbed, and participated actively in every aspect of the procedure.

Chapter 19
Central Lumbar Decompression

Abdel Majid Sheikh Taha, M.D.

COMMON INDICATIONS
- Herniated disc disease
- Spinal stenosis
- Cauda equina syndrome with significant neurological deficit

POSSIBLE COMPLICATIONS
- Wound infection
- Thrombophlebitis
- Dural tears
- Nerve root injury
- Postoperative discitis

ESSENTIAL STEPS
1. General anesthesia
2. Patient positioned proned on Wilson frame
3. Intraoperative fluoroscopy is used to mark level
4. Posterior approach to spine
5. Posterior elements identified
6. Decompression performed (resection of spinal lamina)
7. Nerve roots assessed for stenosis
8. Closure after application of vancomycin powder

OPERATIVE REPORT
Preoperative Diagnosis: Spinal stenosis
Procedure: Central lumbar decompression
Postoperative Diagnosis: Same

S. Saghieh et al. (eds.), *Operative Dictations in Orthopedic Surgery*,
DOI 10.1007/978-1-4614-7479-1_19,
© Springer Science+Business Media New York 2013

Indications: The patient is a ____-year-old M/F who presented with a history of neurologic claudication. The pain-free walking distance is less than one block. After thorough discussion of the surgical procedure, the benefits and the possible complications, the patient opted for surgery.

Description of Operation: Patient was brought to the operating room where he/she was placed supine on the OR stretcher. General anesthesia was administered with endotracheal intubation without difficulty. Prophylactic antibiotics were administered. Foley catheter and appropriate IV lines were placed. Patient was then gently log rolled into position prone on the Wilson frame. Care was taken to protect and pad all pressure points. Fluoroscopy was used to determine the proper levels of stenosis and to draw the incision.

The back was then prepped and draped free in the usual sterile fashion. A midline longitudinal incision was made over the lower lumbar spine. Sharp dissection was carried through subcutaneous tissue, with hemostasis controlled with electrocoagulation. The dorsal tips of the spinous processes were identified. The paraspinal muscles were subperiosteally elevated from the lateral side of the spinous processes. Dissection continued laterally so as to expose the facet joints. A lateral x-ray was taken to assist with level identification. The L_-_and L_-_ facet capsules were identified. The spinous process of L_ was then removed totally. The cranial ½ of the spinous process of L_ and the caudal ½ of the spinous process of L_ were then removed. The dorsal lamina was then thinned with a high-speed burr. Canal entrance was very difficult, secondary to the severe stenosis at the _-_level. The undersurface of the lamina of L_ was finally identified. The ligamentum flavum was markedly thickened, but the lamina of L_ nearly butted against the lamina of L_. Upon entrance into the epidural space, there was complete absence of epidural fat. Decompression continued caudally so as to remove the superior portion of the lamina of L_. The ligamentum flavum where it merged with the medial facet capsule was removed. The thecal sac throughout the surgical procedure was protected with cottonoid patties. An osteotome was utilized to resect the medial 2–3 mm of the inferior facet of L_ bilaterally. A 4 mm Kerrison rongeur removed the markedly thickened medial facet capsule in the medial portion of the superior facet of L_ bilaterally. This greatly freed the lateral recess. L_roots were identified, probed, and found to be free at the end of decompression. The same was repeated for L_ (if other levels were involved).

The wound was then copiously irrigated, including antibiotic irrigant. Patient underwent force of Valsalva maneuver. There was no CSF leak. Soft retaining retractor was removed, and the paraspinal muscles are allowed to fall in their anatomical position. Vancomycin powder was applied. A drain is applied. The supraspinous ligament was reapproximated with multiple Vicryl figure-of-eight sutures. Subcutaneous tissue was closed in layers with 2-0 Vicryl, followed by skin closure with 3-0 Monocryl. Steristrips were applied, followed by a dry sterile dressing.

The patient was then gently log rolled into supine position on the hospital bed, extubated, and taken to the recovery room in satisfactory condition, having tolerated the procedure well. Sponge and needle counts were declared correct×2. Loupe magnification and high intensity illumination were employed throughout the procedure. Estimated blood loss was ___ ml. Postoperative neurologic examination was ___.

Chapter 20
Posterolateral Interspinal Fusion with Pedicle Screws

Joseph G. Khoury, M.D.

COMMON INDICATIONS
- Trauma
- Instability
- Recurrent disk herniations
- Discogenic back pain
- Post-laminectomy instability

POSSIBLE COMPLICATIONS
- Dural tear
- Infection
- Nerve traction injury
- Screw penetration into canal or anteriorly into major vessel
- Graft donor site morbidity

ESSENTIAL STEPS
1. Midline incision.
2. Identify proper level and confirm with x-ray.
3. Dissect subperiosteally down the lamina to the level of the facet joint.
4. Clear facet joint one level cranial but do not strip the capsule off this joint.
5. Continue dissection out laterally at both levels to the tips of the transverse processes.
6. Decorticate the pars and transverse processes.

S. Saghieh et al. (eds.), *Operative Dictations in Orthopedic Surgery*,
DOI 10.1007/978-1-4614-7479-1_20,
© Springer Science+Business Media New York 2013

7. Strip the capsule of the facet joint to be fused and remove cartilage from within the joint.
8. Lay strips of corticocancellous autograft (cancellous side facing ventral) between the transverse processes and along the pars and lamina.
9. Insert pedicle screws.
10. Starting point is at a point where a line down the transverse process intersects a line up the pars.
11. This usually corresponds to the most caudal portion of the superior facet of the level below.
12. Angle in varies depending on the level.
13. Cant c-arm to get a perfect shot down the pedicle and make start point with burr.
14. Continue down pedicle with blunt gear shift confirming position on both views.
15. Do not go beyond half way across the vertebral body on the lateral.
16. Tap the hole.
17. Check for breach of all four walls and the distal part of the hole with feeler.
18. Insert screw.
19. Connect screws depending on type of construct chosen.

OPERATIVE NOTE

Preoperative Diagnosis: Degenerative disk disease L4/L5

Procedure: Posterolateral fusion L4/L5 with autograft bone and pedicle instrumentation

Postoperative Diagnosis: Same

Indications: This patient has loss of disk height on radiographs and a concordant discogram suggesting this location as the source of his pain. He has exhausted all conservative measures and would like to proceed with fusion. He is aware of the risks and the relatively low chance of complete relief and is willing to proceed.

Description of Operation: The patient was properly identified by anesthesia, brought to the operating room, and positioned supine on the cart. General anesthetic was delivered and he was intubated. He was log-rolled onto the Wilson frame. All pressure points were padded. Antibiotics were given. The back was prepped and draped in the usual fashion. A midline incision was made over what was thought to be the L4/L5 level. Once the lumbar fascia was identified, dissection was carried down onto the appropriate level spinous process. A hemostat was placed between the spinous processes of L4 and L5 and its position was confirmed on a lateral radiograph which included the sacrum. Dissection was then carried down the lamina of L4 and L5 bilaterally to the level of the facet joints. The facet capsule of L3/L4 was preserved while the capsule of L4/L5 was stripped. A Cobb elevator and cautery were used to proceed on out to the tips of the transverse processes. A burr was used to decorticate both transverse processes and the pars. The L4/L5 facet joint was also debrided of cartilage with the burr and a curette. Next, the previously harvested corticocancellous autograft was cut into strips and laid down from transverse process to transverse process and across the lamina and pars.

Next attention was directed to the placement of the pedicle screws. We began with the L4 pedicle. The starting point was identified at the juncture of two lines drawn down the transverse process and up the pars. This was at the most inferior portion of the superior facet of L5. The c-arm was used to confirm the correct starting point by tilting the gantry such that the pedicle was seen perfectly on end. The starting point was made with a burr and the pedicle entered with a blunt gear shift. Its position in the center of the pedicle was confirmed on careful biplanar fluoroscopy as the gear shift was advanced. On the lateral, we stopped at the midway point of the vertebral body. The hole was tapped to the same level. A feeler was used to confirm solid superior, inferior, medial, and lateral walls and to confirm the presence of bone at the end of the tunnel. Next the screw was inserted. The remainder of the screws was inserted in the same manner. Finally, the screws were connected with the rod construct and cross-linked. Final radiographs were taken and the wound irrigated. The fascia was closed tightly with interrupted 0-vicryl suture. The subcutaneous layer with a running 2-0 vicryl and the skin with a 3-0 monocryl running subcuticular. A sterile dressing was applied and the patient was turned back into the supine position and awoken from anesthesia.

Chapter 21
Lumbar Anterior Decompression and Fusion with Cage (L2-5)

Abdel Majid Sheikh Taha, M.D.

COMMON INDICATIONS
- Burst fractures
- Instability of the lumbar spine
- Deficiency of vertebral body
- Lesions of vertebral body

POSSIBLE COMPLICATIONS
- Infection
- Nerve injury
- Ureter or large vessel injury

ESSENTIAL STEPS
1. Endotracheal intubation in supine position.
2. Prophylactic antibiotics administered.
3. Position patient in lateral decubitus.
4. Flex table to widen costo-iliac region.
5. Iliac crest bone graft is harvested through posterior approach.
6. Begin incision from between the 11th and 12th ribs extending obliquely towards the lateral margin of the rectus abdominus, midway between the umbilicus and the symphysis.
7. Carefully incise the fascia and fibers of the external, internal obliques, and transverse abdominus muscles.
8. Detach the peritoneum by blunt dissection; take care to not enter the pleural cavity.

S. Saghieh et al. (eds.), *Operative Dictations in Orthopedic Surgery*,
DOI 10.1007/978-1-4614-7479-1_21,
© Springer Science+Business Media New York 2013

9. Retract the abdominal contents with a malleable retractor.
10. Expose the psoas muscle.
11. Identify the genitofemoral nerve and then identify and retract the ureter medially.
12. Palpate the aorta and retract it medially exposing the lateral aspect of the lumbar spine.
13. Identify the sympathetic chain crossing longitudinally and the segmental vessels transversely.
14. Ligate and divide the segmental vessels halfway between the aorta and foramen.
15. Expose all vertebral bodies to be instrumented.
16. Carefully place temporary distraction.
17. Remove disc material from discs above and below involved body.
18. Create trough for cage in vertebral body with burr.
19. Assemble cage and pack with autograft.
20. Place cage and remove distraction device.
21. Size and place lateral plate and screws into vertebral bodies above and below to secure fixation of cage.
22. Carefully close wound reapproximating each layer individually.

OPERATIVE NOTE
Preoperative Diagnosis: Same as above
Procedure: Anterior decompression/corpectomy (mention level), Anterior fusion (mention level)
Postoperative Diagnosis: Same
Description of Operation: The patient was identified as the correct person in the preoperative holding area and was brought into the operative suite. The patient was placed supine on the operative table and the patient identified the operative site and procedure to be done. The patient was then gently induced into general anesthesia and an endotracheal tube was placed. The patient was then repositioned into the right/left lateral decubitus position. An axillary roll was placed and all bony prominences were well padded. The patient was given perioperative antibiotics. The patient was then prepped and draped in the normal sterile fashion.

A posterior longitudinal incision was made over the posterior iliac crest, 2–3 cm lateral to the PSIS. The posterior muscular fascia was then exposed and the fascia was incised in line with the crest, directly over the crest extending down to bone. The outer table of the crest was then exposed with electrocautery, and cobb elevation subperiosteally. The soft tissue was packed away from the bone and an osteotome was utilized to obtain cortical cancellous strips of autograft bone. A currette was then utilized to remove the cancellous bone down to the inner table. Hemostasis was then obtained with bone wax. The periosteum and posterior muscle fascia were then closed in an interrupted fashion as was the subcutaneous tissue. The skin was then closed with an oblique incision and was then made extending from the ... intercostal space posteriorly to the lateral border of the rectus abdominus anteriorly midway between the umbilicus and the pubic symphysis. The external, internal, and transverse abdominal muscles were then incised in line with the incision. Hemostasis was obtained with electrocautery and suture ligature. The peritoneum was carefully detached with blunt dissection from the abdominal wall and the abdominal contents were retracted medially with packing and a malleable retractor. The psoas muscle was then identified and exposed. The genitofemoral nerve was also identified and protected. The ureter was identified and retracted medially. The aorta was then identified, protected, and retracted exposing the vertebral column. The sympathetic chain was identified along with the segmental vessels. The vessels were ligated half way between the aorta and the foramen. The lateral column of the vertebral bodies were cleaned of soft tissue. The disc spaces of the involved lumbar segments of L___ to L ___ were removed with care, palpating the opposite side of the vertebral column. Temporary distraction was placed from L___ to L___. The vertebral body of L__ was then carefully removed from the anterior longitudinal ligament to ___ the posterior longitudinal ligament. Any bone that was determined to be compressing the canal from anteriorly on preoperative films was removed carefully.

The distance between end plates of L__ and L __, bridging the excised body, was measured for sizing of the cage to be used. The appropriate size cage was chosen, assembled, and then packed with previously obtained autograft. Lamina spreaders were used to maintain height in between L__ and L___. The cage was then placed in this space and lamina spreaders were removed. Care was taken to insure the correct placement of the cage. Bone graft was placed anteriorly and laterally but not posteriorly to the cage.

Utilizing the foot plate drill guide for lateral fixation two drill holes were then made in the L__ and L__ vertebral bodies. These were measured and then tapped. Blunt tipped instrumentation screws were then placed. Two rods were then measured, cut, and placed connecting the screws. The locking bolts were seated into position with hand tightening. The wound was irrigated with NS and then closed after all retractors and sponges were removed and sponge and instrument counts were correct. The transverse abdominus, internal, and external oblique musculature were closed in separate layers, in a water tight fashion. The subcutaneous layer was closed in a running water tight fashion and the skin was then closed with ____.

Final sponge count was correct. A sterile dressing was applied. The patient was transferred to the postoperative bed and awakened from general endotracheal anesthesia without incident. The patient was extubated and taken to the post-op recovery room in good condition without evidence of immediate complications. Estimated blood loss was ____.

Dr. _____, was present and scrubbed for the entire procedure.

Chapter 22

Anterior Cervical Decompression and Fusion

Michael J. Huang, M.D.

COMMON INDICATIONS
- Cervical myelopathy from degenerative cervical stenosis
- Herniated nucleus pulposus
- Rheumatoid arthritis

POSSIBLE COMPLICATIONS
- Neurologic damage
- Vascular damage
- Dural tear
- Dysphagia
- Damage to recurrent laryngeal nerve
- Nonunion

ESSENTIAL STEPS:
1. Incision through skin, platysma
2. Identification of carotid sheath as dissection is carried out
3. Deeper dissection to identify esophagus and trachea
4. Further dissection to prevertebral fascia
5. Identification and confirmation of appropriate cervical level(s)
6. Discectomy
7. Measurement of intervertebral disc space and placement of allograft
8. PDGF application

S. Saghieh et al. (eds.), *Operative Dictations in Orthopedic Surgery*,
DOI 10.1007/978-1-4614-7479-1_22,

9. Placement of plate and screws, alignment and fixation confirmation
10. Irrigation, hemostasis, and closure

OPERATIVE NOTE

Preoperative Diagnosis: Cervical myelopathy, central stenosis C5-6, C6-7

Procedure: Anterior cervical discectomy and fusion at C5-6 and C6-7 using bone allograft and plate and screw fixation.

Postoperative Diagnosis: Same

Indications: __-year-old man/woman with worsening evidence of early myelopathy related to cervical spinal stenosis at C5-6 and C6-7. After discussing the risks and benefits of the surgical procedure to decompress and fuse these levels, he/she wished to proceed. Informed consent was obtained.

Description of Operation: The patient was identified by the Anesthesia Team and brought to the main operating room. General anesthetic was administered via the endotracheal tube, and 1 g of Ancef was administered via the IV. The patient was then transferred to the Jackson table where Gardner-Wells tongs were applied. The patient was placed in 7 lb. of traction. The shoulders were taped distally, and the neck was positioned in neutral to slight extension. The patient was then prepped and draped in the standard surgical fashion. Somatosensory evoked potentials were performed throughout the procedure. There was a good wave form, and there were no changes noted by the technician. An anterior approach to the neck was performed from the left side at approximately the level of C5. The skin incision was approximately 5 cm in length. Dissection was carried down through the platysma muscle and just medial to the sternocleidomastoid and carotid sheath. It was carried down lateral to the strap muscles and esophagus. Dissection continued down to the prevertebral fascia, and fluoroscopy was used to localize the levels of C5-6 and C6-7. The interspaces were well visualized, and the anterior aspect of the anulus was removed from first the level of C6-7. The inter-disk material was removed with a pituitary rongeur and curettes. The high-speed burr was used to further prepare the endplates. Large posterior osteophytes were noted at this level, and were undercut with a 2 mm diamond burr. The 4.0 ankle curettes were used to remove the remaining bone with excellent decompression noted at this level.

The wound was copiously irrigated, and good hemostasis was achieved. The interspace measured 6 large. The blood had been previously removed and was prepared with the Symphony platelet concentrating system. The 7 mm large graft was soaked in the platelet concentrate growth factor solution and was impacted into position at C6-7. The AP and lateral fluoroscopy verified the excellent alignment.

Attention was then turned to the next proximal level of C5-6. The interspace was prepared in a similar fashion, taking care to carefully remove the posterior osteophytes and adequately decompress this level as well. After sufficient decompression had been noted, the wound was again thoroughly irrigated, and a 6 large Smith and Nephew graft was impacted into position. Both grafts were in excellent position on both fluoroscopic views. A 41 mm two-segment anterior cervical plate was chosen and positioned across the levels of C5-6 and C6-7. Four screws were placed with standard technique, affixing the plate well. Its position was confirmed with the fluoroscope.

The wound was thoroughly irrigated, and some remaining platelet concentrate was sprinkled in the wound. Excellent hemostasis was noted. The deep cervical fascia was reapproximated with several 2-0 Vicryl interrupted stitches. The platysma was reapproximated using a 2-0 Vicryl interrupted stitch. The subcutaneous tissue was closed with 3-0 Vicryl interrupted stitch. The skin was reapproximated using a running subcuticular 4-0 Monocryl. Steri-Strips were placed, and the wound was covered with sterile 4×4s and a Tegaderm. The Miami J-collar was then placed, and the patient was awakened and extubated and brought to the recovery room in stable condition, with no immediate complications.

Dr. ____ was present and scrubbed for the entire procedure.

Chapter 23

Vertebroplasty

Hamdi G. Sukkarieh, M.D.

COMMON INDICATIONS

- Vertebral compression fractures.
- Osteoporotic fracture refractory to medical therapy.
- Benign or malignant tumor: hemangioma, multiple myeloma, metastatic lesion.
- Osteonecrosis.
- Unstable fractures with movement at wedge deformity.
- Multiple thoracic compression deformities with decreased thoracic cage threatens pulmonary compromise, impacts appetite, GI function, balance.
- Possible structural reinforcement prior to surgical stabilization.

CONTRAINDICATIONS

Absolute Contraindications

- Asymptomatic stable fracture
- Clinically effective medical therapy
- Osteomyelitis of target vertebra
- Uncorrected coagulation disorders
- Acute traumatic fracture of non-osteoporotic vertebra
- Prophylaxis with no evidence of acute fracture
- Allergy to any required component
- Local or systemic infection

S. Saghieh et al. (eds.), *Operative Dictations in Orthopedic Surgery*,
DOI 10.1007/978-1-4614-7479-1_23,
© Springer Science+Business Media New York 2013

Relative Contraindications
- Radicular pain or radiculopathy caused by a compressive syndrome unrelated to vertebral body collapse
- Retropulsed fragment with >20 % spinal canal compromise
- Tumor extension into epidural space
- Severe vertebral body collapse (vertebra plana)
- Stable fracture without pain older than 1 year

POSSIBLE COMPLICATIONS
- Cement leakage
- Neurologic complications
- Pulmonary embolism
- Local pain
- Allergic reaction
- Collapse of adjacent vertebrae after vertebroplasty
- Infection of vertebral body or disc space

ESSENTIAL STEPS
1. Prepping and draping of the back.
2. Inject local anesthetic.
3. Under fluoroscopic guidance, advance needle through skin and subcutaneous tissue, aiming for the pedicle of the desired vertebrae.
4. Advance the needle through the pedicle into the mid vertebral body.
5. Inject desired solutions, followed by methyl methacrylate.
6. Monitor patient for any neurological symptoms.

OPERATIVE NOTE
Preoperative Diagnosis: ___vertebra compression fracture
Procedure: Percutaneous transpedicular ___ vertebroplasty
Postoperative Diagnosis: Same
Indication: This is a ___-year-old M/F with an ___ compression vertebra fracture that is refractory to medical treatment.
Description of Operation: The patient was identified and the site of surgery confirmed. The patient was positioned in the prone position, with all bony prominences padded. The lower back was prepped and draped in the usual sterile fashion. Local anesthetic was applied over the posterolateral access sites. Under fluoroscopic guidance, a 10-gauge vertebroplasty needle was then advanced through the first pedicle of L-- into the mid vertebral body at the

anterior one-third margin. A combination steroid/analgesic/anti-biotic solution was infused into the compressed vertebrae. The patient then underwent vertebroplasty procedure utilizing surgical methyl methacrylate mixed with sterile barium powder for better opacification. Direct fluoroscopy was utilized during the cement injection. The vertebroplasty was performed without difficulty and the needle was subsequently removed. The patient was kept in the prone position for 10 min to allow the cement to harden. The patient did not complain of any significant back pain following the procedure and was neurologically intact.

Postprocedure Care

For the first 24 h after vertebroplasty, bed rest is usually recommended.

Activities may be increased gradually and most regular medications can be resumed.

There may be some soreness for a few days at the puncture site which may be relieved with an ice pack.

Chapter 24

Cervical Laminoplasty

Marc Najjar, M.D.

GOALS OF SURGICAL TREATMENT

- Posterior decompression and reconstruction of the cervical spinal canal

COMMON INDICATIONS

- Multisegmental cervical spondylosis with a narrow canal
- OPLL with continuous or mixed type
- Developmental spinal canal stenosis
- JOA score below 13/17

POSSIBLE COMPLICATIONS

- Maladaptation of the HA spacer to the splitting spinous process: the tip of the spinous process must be cut precisely to accommodate a spacer to the split laminae.
- C5 nerve palsy: in the early postoperative days, pain may occur in the shoulder of the upper arm. After that weakness of the deltoid and the biceps brachii muscles may develop. This palsy is motor-dominant.

ADVANTAGES OF SPINAL PROCESSES MEDIAN SPLITTING LAMINOPLASTY FOR CERVICAL MYELOPATHY

- Short operating time using threaded saw (T-saw) and Hydroxypatite (HA) spacer
- Full expansion of the spinal canal
- Preventing postoperative kyphotic change and the formation of peridural scar tissue
- Nerve root decompression and partial facetectomy
- Spinal stability with bone graft

S. Saghieh et al. (eds.), *Operative Dictations in Orthopedic Surgery*,
DOI 10.1007/978-1-4614-7479-1_24,
© Springer Science+Business Media New York 2013

DISADVANTAGES
- Decreasing ROM of the cervical spine
- Postoperative stiffness in the neck and the interscapular region

CHOOSING LAMINOPLASTY LEVELS
Extent of laminoplasty is usually from C3 to C7. If there is a narrow canal at the C2 level, this level should be included. If an instability is recognized preoperatively, bone grafting for stabilization should be used instead of an HA spacer.

OPERATIVE NOTE
Preoperative Diagnosis: Cervical spondylosis
Procedure: Cervical laminoplasty
Postoperative Diagnosis: Same
Description of Operation:

Positioning: The patient is intubated and placed in the prone position on a four-point supporting frame. Mayfield's pin holder is safe and useful for maintaining cervical alignment in slight extension. In cases of a second operation, the neutral position is better than the extension position so that an airtome can be used instead of a T-saw for splitting of the spinous process. Cervical alignment should be reconfirmed by x-ray before making the skin incision.

Skin Incision: The midline incision is usually made from the C2 spinous process to the T1 spinous process. The ligament nuchae is dissected in midline.

Exposure of the Laminae: The paravertebral muscle is detached from the lamina using an electric cautery, Cobb elevator, and scissors. The semispinal muscles inserted to the C2 lamina are detached bilaterally, making a landmark. The posterior spines from the distal C2 to the proximal T1 are exposed. Each facet is also exposed without injury of the capsule. The edge of each spinous process is cut, and the long spinous process of the C6 and C7 are cut without a fracture of the lamina. The interlaminal soft tissues from the C2-C3 to the C7-T1 are removed with a rongeur and each yellow ligament is exposed.

Median Splitting of the Spinal Process: The epidural space at C2-3 is exposed with removal of the yellow ligament by an air drill and Kerrison rongeur. A cervical intervertebral spreader is useful for exposure of the epidural space at C7-T1. After spreading of the C7-T1 interlaminar space, the median split of the yellow ligament can be found. The yellow ligament is easily removed from this split. The dural membrane is confirmed. The length of the epidural tube is measured from C7-T1 to C2-3. Using an epidural needle (16 gauge), an epidural tube is carefully inserted from the epidural space at C7-T1, and its top is pulled out at the epidural space at C2-3. A T-saw with 0.54-mm diameter is passed through the tube and the T-saw is pulled out. The T-saw runs in the epidural space from C3 to C7. Maintaining cervical lordosis with a lordotic keeper, median splitting of the processes is started from C3 to C7. To avoid generating heat when cutting the bone, physiological saline solution is sprinkled simultaneously. Median splitting is achieved within several minutes. If it is difficult to insert the epidural tube, because of, for example, a severe stenosis, the narrowest interlaminal space should be carefully opened with the same procedure at C7-T1. Median splitting should be separately carried out. If the T-saw is not available, using the thin Kerrison rongeur is recommended to split the remaining spinous processes one by one following the construction of the bilateral gutter.

Constructing the Bilateral Hinge: The line of the lateral gutter is located at the transitional area between the lamina and articular process. Using an air drill with a 4 mm round diamond bur, the outer cortex is cut and thinned. From the cephalad to the caudal direction, each lamina is opened bilaterally with a small curet. Opening the lamina of C7 is achieved after cutting the yellow ligament of C7/T1.

Confirmation of the Decompression: Adhesion between the dura and the yellow ligament is carefully detached with a small elevator. If possible, posterior migration of the spinal cord should be confirmed with an intraoperative ultrasound sonography.

Stabilization of the Hydroxyapatite Spacer: Three-sized spacer trial (12-, 15-, and 20-mm length) is done to determine the width of the spacer. This spacer has small flanges to prevent displacement. A 15-mm spacer is usually used at C3 or C4 and a 20-mm spacer at the lower level. A bilateral bone tunnel for thread suture is made with a 2-mm round diamond bur. A spacer is tightly fixed between the split lamina with two nonabsorbable thread sutures. In case of cervical instability, an iliac bone graft is used for the unstable segment instead of an HA spacer, and bone chips are placed on the bilateral gutter.

Reattachment of the Semispinal Muscle: The semispinal cervical muscles are securely reattached to the spinous process of the axis bilaterally. This procedure prevents a postoperative malalignment of the cervical spine, especially kyphotic change.

Closure: A suction drainage tube is placed on the laminae and the wound is closed layer by layer. Postoperative lateral x-ray shows normal sagittal alignment. CT scan shows adequate spinal decompression.

Pitfalls:

■ Making a lateral gutter outside occurs in facet fusion.

■ Using a T-saw may damage the spinal cord on the flexion position.

■ Beware of stabilization of the HA spacer in case of a fragile lateral gutter. A too-tight thread suture may destroy the lateral gutter.

Postoperative Care: A suction drainage tube is removed within 24 h. Sitting and walking is permitted with a Philadelphia collar for 2 weeks. 3 weeks postoperatively, isometric exercises of the neck and shoulder is started, and a soft collar is used. 5 weeks postoperatively, the soft collar is removed. Early muscle exercises are recommended to maintain ROM of the neck. Postoperative stiffness in the neck and shoulder resolves within 12 months.

Part III

Pelvis, Hip, and Thigh

Chapter 25
Hybrid Total Hip Arthroplasty

Rida Adel Kassim, M.D.

COMMON INDICATIONS
- Osteoarthritis (primary and secondary)
- Inflammatory arthritis (rheumatoid, ankylosing spondylitis, etc.)
- Avascular necrosis
- Complex fractures (acetabular and femoral neck)

POSSIBLE EARLY COMPLICATIONS
- Infection
- Fracture
- Dislocation
- Leg length discrepancy
- Pulmonary Embolus
- Deep vein thrombosis
- Neurovascular injury

POSSIBLE LATE COMPLICATIONS
- Aseptic loosening
- Osteolysis
- Septic loosening

ESSENTIAL STEPS
1. Lateral Decubitus positioning with great care to protect nonoperative extremities
2. Isolation of the Perineum using Steridrape
3. Posterolateral Kocher-Langenbach incision
4. Slit the iliotibial band and the fibers of the gluteus maximus

S. Saghieh et al. (eds.), *Operative Dictations in Orthopedic Surgery*,
DOI 10.1007/978-1-4614-7479-1_25,
© Springer Science+Business Media New York 2013

5. Release the gluteal sling and cauterize the first perforator
6. Release the short external rotators
7. Medial-based posterior capsular flap
8. Dislocate the hip and osteotomize the femoral neck slightly longer than expected
9. Exposure of the acetabulum with removal of medial osteophyte
10. Must visualize the pulvinar fat and the cotyloid notch
11. Ream 1 mm less than the final implant and insert implant with 1–2 screws
12. Acetabular orientation should be 20° anteversion and 45° lateral opening
13. Obtain access to the femoral canal posterolaterally to avoid varus
14. Clear loose cancellous bone from the proximal femur
15. Broach and trial the femoral component (20° femoral anteversion)
16. Irrigate and dry the canal
17. Place cement restrictor and cement plug
18. Pressurize the cement in the doughy phase
19. Insert femoral stem with care not to go in varus
20. Repair the capsule and short external rotators through bone tunnels
21. Layered closure over drains

OPERATIVE NOTE

This is a ___-year-old patient who has been complaining of R/L hip pain for the past ___ years.

Radiographs showed severe arthritis of the hip with complete destruction of the joint.

The patient had—intraarticular steroid injection with no improvement.

Preoperative Diagnosis: R/L hip arthritis

Procedure: L/R total hip arthroplasty state the implant you used

Postoperative Diagnosis: Same

Operative Procedure: The patient was identified and the correct operative extremity confirmed. The patient was brought in the operating room and spinal or general anesthetic was administered. Antibiotic was administered intravenously. The patient was then placed in the left lateral decubitus position using a peg-board for positioning. The anterior pelvis peg was placed at the level of the pubic symphysis and the posterior peg was placed superior to the gluteal cleft. The position of the pelvis relative to the floor was evaluated and confirmed to be perpendicular. A bolster was placed along the lateral chest wall on the down side to protect the axilla. The down arm was padded with a pillow to the level of the shoulder in approximately 60° of shoulder flexion and neutral abduction. The down elbow was then flexed to 45° and supported with pillows. The upside arm is relaxed on a stirrup in a 90/90 position; care to the elbow is undertaken. The nonoperative lower extremity was padded to protect the peroneal nerve and bony prominences. An impervious drape was placed with to isolate the perineum. The operative leg was then prepped with iodine gel from the ankle to the pelvis and draped with an impervious U-drape followed by impervious hip drapes. Circumferential iodine impregnated self-adherent film was then applied.

A posterolateral approach (Modified Kocher-Langenbach) was utilized starting approximately 8 cm distal to the greater trochanter along the anterior third of the femoral shaft extending proximally over the greater trochanter at the mid point and continuing approximately 6 cm proximal curving slightly posterior in line with the gluteus maximus fibers. The incision was carried through the subcutaneous tissue to the iliotibial band. The iliotibial band was incised distally and extended proximally in-line with the skin incision. The gluteus maximus fibers were bluntly spread with finger dissection while hemostasis was maintained. The gluteal sling was identified and incised 1 cm from the insertion onto the femur with the underlying sciatic nerve protected with a hemostat. The first perforator was identified and cauterized. The Charnley retractor was placed taking care to ensure protection of the sciatic nerve. The interval between the gluteus minimus and the capsule was identified and Homan retractor was placed on the superior aspect of the femoral neck. Extreme care was used to prevent excessive retraction on the hip abductors. The piriformis tendon was identified and incised off the insertion in the piriformis fossa. The remaining external rotators were then identified (conjoined tendon, obturator externis, and quadratus femoris) and incised off of their insertion into the greater trochanter. The lesser trochanter was visualized. To create a medially based posterior capsular flap a curved Beaver blade was placed onto the superior aspect of the acetabular rim and the capsule was incised laterally to the neck of the femur at the 12 o'clock position. A Homan retractor was placed on the inferior aspect of the femoral neck and the soft tissues retracted posteriorly allowing placement of the curved blade on the inferior rim of the acetabulum. The inferior capsule was incised from the acetabular rim laterally to the femoral neck. The capsule was then reflected off the posterior aspect of the neck from the 12 o'clock to the 6 o'clock position completing the medial-based posterior capsular flap and exposing the femoral head. The estimated center of the femoral head was marked with and the distance from the superior aspect of the lesser trochanter to the center of the femoral head was measured. The femoral head was dislocated by a combined hip flexion, adduction, and internal rotation. Examination of the femoral head revealed the patient had marked erosive changes in the femoral head as well as osteophytes. There was marked flattening of the femoral head. The femoral head was then osteotomized at approximately 22 mm above the lesser trochanter.

The acetabulum was then exposed using four retractors (anterior acetabular retractor placed over the anterior rim, Steinman pin placed into the superior ilium retracting the abductors, curved cobra retractor into the obturator foramen, and posterior acetabular retractor placed between the labrum and posterior capsule on the posterior rim). Examination revealed the acetabulum to be slightly shallow and in addition there were erosive changes in addition to anterior and posterior osteophytes. The remaining labrum was then incised off the rim with a straight blade in a circumferential fashion. The obturator retractor was repositioned. The acetabulum was reamed starting with a 42 mm perpendicular to the floor to remove the medial osteophyte and expose the pulvinar 49 mm and was enlarged to the size template or when we reach bleeding one with biequatorial catch. Hemispherical cup was placed with approximately 45° of lateral opening and 20° of anteversion. The anterior and posterior osteophytes were removed with a curved osteotome and the ischium and pubis were palpated to confirm correct positioning of the cup. Two acetabular screws were place in the posterior–superior and posterior–inferior quadrants. The trial acetabular liner was screwed into place.

The retractors were then removed and the hip was brought into flexion, adduction, and internal rotation (with the leg directed perpendicular to the ceiling). All remaining soft tissue was removed from the piriformis fossa. The entry site for the canal instrumentation was identified on the posterolateral aspect of the femoral neck. A chisel box osteotome was used to open the medullary canal laterally into the base of the trochanter. The T-handle starter broach was used to enter the medullary canal followed by the Christmas tree reamer to remove weak cancellous bone. Rasping of the femur was done sequential taking good care for version. Calcar reamer was used to clean the neck cut. A trial reduction was performed and hip was evaluated for stability (anterior stability checked with combined extension and external rotation in 30° and posterior stability checked with combined flexion to 100°, internal rotation to 40°, and adduction to 30°). Trial components were removed.

The final acetabular polyethylene liner was inserted. The femur was irrigated mechanically. An adequate size cement restrictor was placed at a depth to allow a 2 cm distal cement mantle. The cement was mixed. The cement was centrifuged for approximately 90 s and then a cement gun pressurizer was used to inject the cement in the canal in the doughy stage. The femoral component was then placed into the femoral canal in approximately 20° of anteversion. Final trial was done for the head neck size. Reduction with adequate head size was performed. Drill holes were placed through the greater trochanter and the external rotators were sewn to the capsule through these bone tunnels using #1 vicryl suture. The gluteal sling was also reapproximated with #1 vicryl suture. A final irrigation was performed with antibiotic loaded normal saline. Two deep drains were placed deep to the tensor fascia. The IT band was closed with #1 vicryl. #0 vicryl was used for the subcutaneous closure and skin with stapler. Adaptec, fluffs, and 8 in. bias wrap dressing were applied. The patient was placed supine on the bed while maintaining total hip precautions. The patient was taken to the recovery room where x-rays were obtained confirming reduction after transfer.

Chapter 26

Primary Uncemented Total Hip Arthroplasty

Rola H. Rashid, M.D.

COMMON INDICATIONS
- Severely symptomatic hip osteoarthritis

POSSIBLE COMPLICATIONS
- Risks of anesthesia
- Infection
- Thromboembolic phenomenon
- Neurocirculatory compromise
- Fracture dislocation
- Stiffness
- Leg length inequality
- Late loosening

ESSENTIAL STEPS
1. Patient positioning
2. Incision
3. Identifying and tagging short external rotators
4. Opening and tagging capsule
5. Femoral neck cut
6. Acetabular exposure
7. Excision of labrum
8. Reaming of acetabulum
9. Placement of acetabular shell
10. Placement of liner
11. Preparation of femur

S. Saghieh et al. (eds.), *Operative Dictations in Orthopedic Surgery*,
DOI 10.1007/978-1-4614-7479-1_26,
© Springer Science+Business Media New York 2013

12. Assess leg length and stability
13. Placement of femoral component and femoral head
14. Wound closure

OPERATIVE NOTE

Preoperative Diagnosis: Severe hip degenerative joint disease
Procedure: Total hip arthroplasty
Postoperative Diagnosis: Same
Description of Operation: The patient was brought into the operating room and placed in the supine position. After induction of general anesthesia, prophylactic antibiotics were given. A Foley catheter was sterilely placed. The patient was placed in the left lateral decubitus position on a Capello positioner. All extremities were well padded. The appropriate leg was prepped and draped for surgery. An incision was carried out starting 4–5 cm above the greater trochanter and slightly posteriorly, going over the greater trochanter, and distally over the lateral shaft of the femur for 6 cm. The incision was carried through the subcutaneous tissue and iliotibial band. The Charnley retractor was placed. A Hohmann was placed between capsule and gluteus minimus. The piriformis, conjoint tendon, obturator externus, and quadratus femoris were incised off their insertion into the proximal femur. A medially based posterior acetabular flap was made in the capsule. The femoral head was dislocated. Examination of the femoral head and synovium was performed. The femoral neck was osteotomized __mm above the lesser trochanter as templated. The labrum was excised. The acetabulum was sequentially reamed to the appropriate diameter. A trial component was placed in approximately 40° of lateral opening and 20° of anteversion. It showed good fit. The appropriate final component was press fit into the acetabulum. Two domed screws were placed to secure the fixation. The anterior and posterior osteophytes of the acetabulum were removed and the trial liner with an appropriately sized inner diameter was placed. This was a neutral liner. The femur was flexed and internally rotated to 90°. A jaws retractor was placed anteriorly, a curved cobra was placed medially, and a bent Hohmann was placed laterally. A cookie cutter followed by a T-bar reamer and pilot hole reamer were used. The femoral canal was sequentially reamed to the appropriate diameter. The broach was placed in approximately 10–15° of anteversion. The calcar was reamed. The appropriately sized neck was placed on the broach as well as the trial head of __ mm in diameter. The hip was located. Range of motion was measured and found to be acceptable. X-ray was taken and showed good position of the trials with no evidence

of fractures. The leg length appeared equal. All the trial components were removed. The acetabular shell was exposed, irrigated, and the liner was impacted into the shell being sure as to have no soft tissue interposition. The femur was once again exposed. The femoral component was placed with appropriate scratch fit and anteversion. After seating the component on the calcar, the trunnion was cleaned, the head was twisted onto the trunnion, and then was impacted into place with a mallet. The femoral head was relocated into the acetabular liner being sure as to have no soft tissue interposition. The external rotators and capsule were reapproximated to the greater trochanter through drill holes. A drain was placed deep to the IT band coming through the anterolateral skin. #1 running PDS was used for IT band closure. #1 PDS in two layers was used for subcutaneous closure. The skin was closed with staples. A sterile dressing was applied. The patient was placed supine, placed on the hospital bed, and taken to the recovery room in satisfactory condition.

There were no immediate complications noted.

A Staff member was present and scrubbed for the entire procedure.

Chapter 27
Revision Hip Arthroplasty

Rida Adel Kassim, M.D.

COMMON INDICATIONS
- Aseptic loosening of the femoral or acetabular component, or both
- Periprosthetic fracture
- Progressive osteolysis
- Recurrent dislocation
- Infection

POSSIBLE EARLY COMPLICATIONS
- Infection
- Dislocation
- Fracture
- Pulmonary embolism
- Deep vein thrombosis
- Neurovascular Injury
- Dislocation
- Leg length discrepancy

POSSIBLE LATE COMPLICATIONS
- Nonunion of femoral osteotomy
- Loosening
- Osteolysis

ESSENTIAL STEPS
1. Lateral decubitus positioning
2. Padding of the axilla, elbow, and the knee on the unoperated side
3. Isolation of perineum with steridrape

S. Saghieh et al. (eds.), *Operative Dictations in Orthopedic Surgery*,
DOI 10.1007/978-1-4614-7479-1_27,

4. Posterolateral Kocher-Langenbach incision
5. Separate the iliotibial band from the vastus lateralis fascia
6. Skeletonize the femur
7. Decision and exposure by either
   (a) Maintain trochanter
   (b) Standard trochanter osteotomy
   (c) Trochanter slide or
   (d) Extended trochanter osteotomy
8. Capsulotomy with exposure of both acetabular column
9. Removal of the femoral component
   (a) Extended osteotomy distal to the cement mantle or prosthesis
   (b) cortical window
10. Ream 1 mm less than the final implant and insert implant with dome screws
11. Acetabular orientation should be 20° anteversion and 45° lateral opening
12. Minimum of 4–5 cm scratch fit when using extensively coated femoral stems
13. Repair the capsule and short external rotators through bone tunnels
14. Layered closure over drains

OPERATIVE NOTE

This is a ___-year-old patient who had a R/L total hip replacement ___ years ago. He/she started experiencing mechanical type of pain over the past years that has increased tremendously. Radiographs were in favor of loosening of both components.

Preoperative Diagnosis: Failed L/R total hip

Procedure: Revision total hip arthroplasty (L/R) with the type of implant used

Postoperative Diagnosis: Same

Operative Procedure: The patient was identified and the correct operative extremity confirmed. He/she was brought in the operating room and a combined spinal and epidural anesthetic or general anesthesia was performed. Antibiotics were administered intravenously. A Foley catheter was placed under sterile conditions. He/she was then placed in the lateral decubitus position using a peg-board for positioning. The anterior pelvis peg was placed at the level of the pubic symphysis and the posterior peg was placed superior to the gluteal cleft. The position of the pelvis relative to the floor was evaluated and confirmed to be perpendicular. A bolster was placed along the lateral chest wall on the down side to protect the axilla. The upside arm relaxed over a stirrup in a 90/90 position with a care to pad the elbow region. The down arm was padded with a pillow to the level of the shoulder in approximately 60° of shoulder flexion and neutral abduction. The down elbow was then flexed to 45° and supported with pillows. The nonoperative lower extremity was padded to protect the peroneal nerve and bony prominences. An impervious drape was placed to isolate the perineum. The operative leg was then prepped with iodine gel from the ankle to the pelvis and draped with an impervious U-drape followed by impervious hip drapes. Circumferential iodine impregnated self-adherent film was then applied.

The old incision was a posterolateral approach and it was utilized for the revision exposure. The old scar was removed in an elliptical fashion incorporating the new incision starting approximately 10 cm distal to the greater trochanter along the anterior third of the femoral shaft extending proximally over the greater trochanter at the mid point and continuing approximately 6–7 cm proximal curving slightly posterior in line with the gluteus maximus fibers. The incision was carried through the subcutaneous tissue to the iliotibial band. The iliotibial band was incised distally in an area of unscarred tissue. The interval between the vastus lateralis and the iliotibial band was identified. This interval was developed proximally along the anterior and posterior flaps. The gluteus maximus fibers were bluntly spread with finger dissection while hemostasis was maintained. The gluteal sling was identified and incised 1 cm from the insertion onto the femur with the underlying sciatic nerve protected with a hemostat. The first perforator was identified and cauterized. Towels were sewn to the iliotibial band anteriorly and posteriorly to isolate the skin flaps from the wound. The Charnley retractor was placed taking care to ensure protection of the sciatic nerve. With blunt finger dissection the anterior and posterior margins of the gluteus medius were identified. The decision was made to perform an extended trochanteric osteotomy for removal of the femoral component. The interval between the gluteus minimus and the capsule was identified and Homan retractor was placed on the superior aspect of the femoral neck. Extreme care was used to prevent excessive retraction on the hip abductors. The piriformis and the remaining short external rotators of the hip were scarred to the posterior capsule and this whole layer was elevated as a medially based flap starting superiorly and extending along the posterior aspect of the greater trochanter to the junction of the prosthesis and remaining femoral neck. The proximal femur was skeletonized to the level of the lesser trochanter in a subperiosteal fashion using the cautery. The junction between the remaining proximal femur and the prosthesis was developed circumferentially with alternating cautery and rounger. Patient had a large amount of histiocytosis in the joint with granulomatous disease. We took one culture from the hip and sent fluid for a cell count. With the femoral head within the acetabulum, the granulomatous tissue and the capsule were removed with alternating cautery and rounger in order to mobilized the articulation and visualize the entire margin of the acetabular component. Extreme care was taken to prevent excess retraction on the posterior soft tissue.

The extended trochanteric osteotomy was then performed starting at the posterior base or the greater trochanter. A pencil tip pneumatic drill was used to create sequential perforations distally in a longitudinal fashion ending approximately 5 cm distal to vastus lateralis ridge. This posterior margin of the extended osteotomy was just anterior to the linea aspera. A sagittal saw was then used to complete the longitudinal corticotomy. At the distal aspect of the osteotomy a Cobb was used to gently elevate the vastus lateralis to expose the anterolateral third of the femur at this level (care was taken to maintain the soft tissue attachments to the proximal fragment). The pencil tip burr was used to extend the osteotomy anteriorly one-third the circumference of the femur beveling superiorly. At the anterior portion of the distal aspect of the osteotomy, the corticotomy was extended proximally for 5–6 mm to prevent extension of the osteotomy distally. The anterior–proximal aspect of the osteotomy (the anterior base of the greater trochanter) was cleared of soft tissue and short corticotomy was made with the pencil tip burr for a length of 5–6 mm. Several wide osteotomes were then used to elevate the extended osteotomy fragment anteriorly with the anterior-based hinge leaving the remaining 2/3rd tube of proximal femur intact. The proximal portion of the broken femoral stem was visualized and removed. The remaining cement was thinned with a burr; the distal mantle was drilled and removed with handheld cement removal instruments. Using a cable passer, a cable was placed around the femur just distal to the osteotomy site to prevent propagation during the femoral preparation.

The polyethylene from the loose acetabular component was removed by drilling 3.2 mm hole in the center portion and screwing a 6.5 mm fully threaded cancellous screw into the polyethylene causing dislodgement of the liner. The acetabular screw was removed and the loose acetabular cup retrieved. The acetabulum was then exposed using four retractors (anterior acetabular retractor placed over the anterior rim, Steinman pin placed into the superior ilium retracting the abductors, curved cobra retractor into the obturator foramen, and posterior acetabular retractor). A debridement was performed and the columns evaluated and found to be intact. The acetabulum was reamed. Care was taken not to remove excess bone and to only ream to viable bone. A hemispherical cup was placed with approximately 45° of lateral opening and 20° of anteversion and three acetabular dome screws were placed. The trial acetabular liner was screwed into place. In case of severe bone deficiencies in the acetabulum with pelvic discontinuity, we resort to the use of either rings or cages with cemented poly-liner.

The retractors were then removed and the hip was brought into flexion, adduction, and internal rotation (with the leg directed perpendicular to the ceiling). Based on our preoperative templating, we began remaining the femoral canal with the 7 mm straight reamer and continuing up to the size template or until the reamer is cleaning viable bone. Afterward we begin rasping till the size needed with caring for adequate version. Trial reduction performed with assessment for leg length and stability. The trial components were then removed and the acetabulum exposed. The final acetabular liner was impacted in place after irrigation was performed. The femur was then flexed, adducted, and internally rotated so the leg was perpendicular to the ceiling. The canal was irrigated and the final component was inserted with 10–20° of anteversion. There was 5 cm of scratch-fit. The tapers were cleaned and dried and the final femoral head with neck was placed and impacted. The acetabulum was then irrigated and the hip reduced under direct visualization. Two cables were placed around the proximal femur and the trochanteric fragment. Drill holes were placed through the greater trochanter and the external rotators were sewn to the capsule through these bone tunnels using #1 nonabsorbable suture. The gluteal sling was also reapproximated with #1 nonabsorbable suture. A final irrigation was performed with antibiotic loaded normal saline. Two deep drains were placed deep to the tensor fascia. The IT band was closed using #1 Vicryl. #0 Vicryl was used for the subcutaneous closure and the skin with stapler. Adaptic, fluffs, and 8 in. bias wrap dressing were applied. The patient was placed supine put on the bed while maintaining total hip precautions. The patient was taken to the recovery room where x-rays were obtained confirming reduction after transfer.

Chapter 28
Core Decompression

Said Saghieh, M.D.

COMMON INDICATIONS
- Early stages of avascular necrosis of the femoral head

POSSIBLE COMPLICATIONS
- Wound infection
- Osteomyelitis
- Proximal femur fracture
- Penetration of the articular cartilage
- Progression of the disease

ESSENTIAL STEPS
1. Careful preoperative assessment (history, physical examination, radiographic and MRI staging).
2. Positioning on a fracture table.
3. Assure obtaining good images under fluoroscopic guidance before draping.
4. Introduction of the guiding pin to the involved area.
5. Reaming.
6. Anatomic closure of incision.

OPERATIVE NOTE
Preoperative Diagnosis: Avascular necrosis of the femoral head
Procedure: Core Decompression
Postoperative Diagnosis: Same
Indications: ___ yo male/female who presented with hip pain of ____ months duration and was diagnosed with avascular necrosis of the femoral head based on the imaging studies.

S. Saghieh et al. (eds.), *Operative Dictations in Orthopedic Surgery*,
DOI 10.1007/978-1-4614-7479-1_28,
© Springer Science+Business Media New York 2013

Description of Operation: The patient and surgical site were identified and marked. The patient underwent anesthesia per the anesthesia team. The patient was positioned supine on the fracture table with the involved hip in zero degree of extension and 15° of internal rotation. The contralateral lower extremity was abducted with the hip and the knee flexed. The image intensifier was brought in between the two lower extremities. Good visualization of the femoral head was confirmed on both anteroposterior and lateral views.

IV antibiotics were administered. The extremity was prepped and draped from the iliac crest to the lower thigh in the usual sterile fashion.

A 2 cm skin incision was performed on the midlateral aspect of the thigh two fingers breadth distal to the greater trochanter. The fascia lata was split longitudinally. Under fluoroscopy control a 3.2-mm threaded guide pin was inserted through the lateral cortex just proximal to the level of the lesser trochanter into the area of necrosis. The tip of the guide pin was directed to the center of the diseased segment of the bone as seen on the preoperative MRI. Its final position was checked with the image intensifier in the AP, lateral, and oblique planes. There was no penetration of the articular surface.

Then an 8 mm hollow coring device was inserted over the guide pin through the cortical window and advanced under fluoroscopy guidance to within a few millimeters of the subchondral plate. Core specimen was retrieved and sent for histology examination.

Wound was irrigated and closed in anatomical layers; the fascia with 0-vicryl, the subcutaneous tissue with 2-0 vicryl, and the skin with 4-0 monocryl in subcuticular fashion. Sterile dressing was applied.

Post-op regimen: Protective weight bearing for 6 weeks.

No intraoperative complications.

Staff was present and scrubbed for entire procedure.

Chapter 29
Femoral Antegrade IM Nail

Ziad Elkhoury, M.D.

COMMON INDICATIONS
- Femoral shaft fracture

POSSIBLE COMPLICATIONS
- Infection
- Nonunion
- Malunion
- Hardware failure
- Limb length discrepancy (especially shortening)

ESSENTIAL STEPS
1. Position patient on fracture table
2. Obtain reduction
3. Identify entry point
4. Ream entry point
5. Pass ball-tipped guide wire
6. Ream canal
7. Determine the proper nail length
8. Exchange of the guide wire
9. Insert nail (determine proper length)
10. Proximal and distal locking screws

OPERATIVE NOTE
Indication: This is a young patient who was hit by a car and was transferred to the emergency room with an isolated femur fracture, R/L.

Preoperative Diagnosis: Femoral shaft fracture (describe level, site, pattern, open or closed)

S. Saghieh et al. (eds.), *Operative Dictations in Orthopedic Surgery*,
DOI 10.1007/978-1-4614-7479-1_29,

Procedure: Closed reduction and intramedullary antegrade nail fixation

Postoperative Diagnosis: Same

Description of Operation: The patient was identified and the surgical site was marked in the preholding area. The patient was transported to the operating room, and positioned supine for induction of anesthetic. General anesthesia was induced by the anesthesiologist. The patient was positioned supine in banana shape on the fracture table using boot traction. All pressure points were well padded. Pre-op IV antibiotics (list name and dose) were administered. The (Right or Left) buttock and lower extremity were prepped and draped in a sterile fashion. Closed reduction of the fracture was achieved under fluoroscopy guidance. A 4 cm oblique skin incision was made proximal to the tip of the greater trochanter. Electrocautery was used to dissect through the subcutaneous tissues. Gluteus maximus fascia was incised in line with the skin incision. Blunt dissection was used to reach the bone. The threaded guide pin was placed in the appropriate position in the piriformis fossa (or the tip of greater trochanter) using fluoroscopic guidance. A cannulated reamer was used to ream the nail entry site over the threaded guide wire, followed by insertion of the perforated awl. The awl and the guide pin were then removed. Under fluoroscopic guidance, the ball-tipped guide was inserted into the femoral canal, across the fracture site, to the physeal scar distally. The canal was reamed, starting with 8 mm reamer up to size (insert size). Nail length was then assessed. Exchange of the ball-tipped guide by a smooth tipped one was done with the help of a plastic sheath. Traction was released. A (diameter and size) nail was placed on the appropriate nail guide, and carefully inserted into the femoral canal. Fracture reduction and nail position were confirmed with fluoroscopy. The proximal guide was used to drill and place one proximal locking screw. Then the nail introducer assembly was removed. The C-arm was repositioned to identify one of the distal nail holes as a perfect circle on the lateral view. The drill bit was tapped into the bone so it obscured the perfect circle, then it was drilled across the hole. Using the depth gauge, screw length was determined, and the screw was placed. Proper screw placement was confirmed using fluoroscopy. The same procedure was repeated for the second distal interlocking screws. Finally, the proximal end cap was inserted. The wounds were irrigated. The fascia was closed with vicryl 0 and subcutaneous tissues were closed with vicryl 2.0. Skin was closed with staples. A sterile dressing was applied. The patient was awakened from anesthesia and was transported to the recovery room in satisfactory condition. There were no immediate complications associated with the procedure.

A staff was present and scrubbed in during the procedure.

Chapter 30

Femoral Neck Fracture Closed Reduction and Percutaneous Multiple Screw Fixation

Anthony V. Mollano, M.D.

COMMON INDICATIONS

- Femoral neck fractures (displaced or nondisplaced) in active adults, including active elderly, ideal when good bone quality is present.

POSSIBLE COMPLICATIONS

- Mortality (multifactorial)
- Infection (1–16 %)
- Thromboembolism (high risk)
- Pressure sores (30 % if debilitated)
- Loss of fixation
- Avascular necrosis (4–40 %)
- Nonunion (2–22 %)
- Screw penetration of the femoral head
- Subtrochanteric fracture at screw sites

ESSENTIAL STEPS

1. Administer anesthesia (general, regional/spinal, or even local in a cooperative patient).
2. Transfer patient to fracture table compatible with fluoroscopy.

S. Saghieh et al. (eds.), *Operative Dictations in Orthopedic Surgery*,
DOI 10.1007/978-1-4614-7479-1_30,
© Springer Science+Business Media New York 2013

3. In undisplaced fractures not requiring reduction, position the affected hip in neutral abduction, in neutral flexion-extension, and in sufficient internal rotation bringing the femoral neck parallel to floor.

4. Most displaced fractures could be reduced with closed techniques; the Leadbetter technique involves manipulation of affected hip in flexion at 90°, and the Whitman technique involves traction on the limb in extension, followed by internal rotation in extension and abduction, followed by abduction and internal rotation.

5. Attain anatomic reduction (acceptable angulation: 130–150° of valgus on AP, and less than 15° of anterior or posterior angulation on lateral).

6. After sterile prep, some place a radiopaque K-wire guide through the skin in two places on anterior aspect of hip in-line with the femoral neck.

7. Incise over proximal femur down to fascia lata.

8. Insert three or four guide-pins, staying within central 2/3 of the femoral head.

9. Loosen traction and impact fracture by pounding over greater trochanter under fluoroscope.

10. Measure screw length, insert cannulated self-tapping lag screw (6–7 mm diameter) with washer (to prevent lateral cortex penetration), so that screw tip remains at least 7 mm away from sub-chondral bone; then remove guide pins (one at a time prior to next screw placement).

11. Irrigate wound, close in layers, and obtain AP and lateral radiographs (before breaking sterile field).

OPERATIVE NOTE

Preoperative Diagnosis: Femoral neck fracture

Procedure: Closed reduction and internal fixation, femoral neck fracture

Postoperative Diagnosis: Same

Indications: This is an *X*-year-old osteoporotic patient ambulator who fell today and suffered a femoral neck fracture. He/she is unable to bear weight. The patient understood the risks and benefits of surgery, and elected to proceed.

Description of Operation: The patient was brought to the operating room, placed supine on the operating table, and a spinal anesthetic was delivered. He/she was then moved onto the fracture table. Fluoroscopy was brought in, and the fracture was reduced. The patient was prepped and draped in a sterile fashion. A 5.0 cm incision was made over the proximal femur, and carried down sharply down to the fascia lata, which was incised in-line with the skin incision. Blunt dissection was utilized to come down onto the proximal femur. Hemostasis was attained. Under fluoroscopic guidance, four guide wires from the cannulated system were inserted: one was in the inferior center position, one was in the proximal anterior position, one was in proximal posterior position, and the other one superior middle. Traction was let off and the hip was rotated to fluoroscopically confirm placement of all pins outside of the hip joint. The screws were measured, sequentially drilled, and inserted under fluoroscopic guidance. The fracture was then copiously irrigated with normal saline, the fascia lata was closed with #1 Vicryl, the subcutaneous layer with 2-0 Vicryl, the skin was stapled, and a sterile dressing was applied. There were no complications. Blood loss was minimal. The patient was sent to the recovery room in stable condition. Sponge, needle, and instrument counts were correct. The Attending Staff Surgeon was present, scrubbed, and participated actively in all aspects of the procedure.

Chapter 31

Intertrochanteric Open Reduction and Internal Fixation with Dynamic Hip Screw

Moustapha Awada, M.D.

COMMON INDICATIONS

- Stable and unstable intertrochanteric fractures
- Some of femur neck fractures (base of neck)

POSSIBLE COMPLICATIONS

- Loss of fixation in <10 % of cases, most often with unstable fracture pattern
- Malunion
- Nonunion
- DVT/Pulmonary embolism
- Superficial or deep infection

ESSENTIAL STEPS

1. Patient position on fracture table
2. Fracture reduction under fluoroscopy
3. Incision, exposure of the bone
4. Guide pin placement
5. Fixation
6. Closure

OPERATIVE NOTE

Indications: The patient is a ___-year-old F/M who sustained a trauma to R/L hip resulting in stable/unstable intertrochanteric fracture. The patient and his/her family elected to proceed with

S. Saghieh et al. (eds.), *Operative Dictations in Orthopedic Surgery*,
DOI 10.1007/978-1-4614-7479-1_31,
© Springer Science+Business Media New York 2013

surgical fixation after discussion of the risks and the benefits of the procedure.

Preoperative Diagnosis: L/R intertrochanteric hip fracture

Procedure: Open reduction internal fixation of R/L intratrochanteric hip fracture with dynamic hip screw and sideplate

Postoperative Diagnosis: Same

Description of Operation: The patient was identified in the preoperative holding area and brought to the operating room. Epidural/general anesthetic was given. Patient was transferred onto the operative fracture-table carefully. The non-injured leg was placed in a well-padded leg holder. The injured leg was placed in the traction unit with the foot well padded. All other pressure points were also well padded. IV antibiotics (name and dose) were administered. Closed reduction was performed under fluoroscopy control. This was obtained by applying longitudinal traction on the abducted and externally rotated hip. The hip was then adducted to neutral and external rotation deformity was corrected to neutral. Near anatomic alignment of the fracture was noted on the fluoroscopy in the AP and lateral views.

The affected lower extremity was prepped and draped in the normal sterile fashion. Fluoroscopy was used to mark the site of best skin incision.

A 7–8 cm incision was made longitudinally over the lateral aspect of the proximal thigh starting proximally at the flare of the greater trochanter. The subcutaneous tissues and the fascia lata were dissected with a cautery. The vastus lateralis fascia was incised in L shape fashion. A Cobb elevator was used to dissect the vastus lateralis muscle off the lateral aspect of the femur. A 135° guide was used to introduce the guide pin in the center of the femoral neck. Once this was confirmed on the AP and lateral views, the threaded pin was advanced through the femoral neck into the femoral head. It stopped in the subchondral bone, 10 mm away of the articular surface. The intraosseous distance was measured and the triple reamer was set adequately to ream over the guide pin. Then the triple reamer was removed and tapping was performed over the guide pin.

The appropriate size hip screw was then inserted. Adequate central positioning with its tip at 10 mm from the articular surface was noted on the AP and lateral views. An x-hole side plate was placed over the central pin to be assembled to the hip screw and laid flush against the femoral shaft. ___ 4.5 cortical screws were placed under fluoroscopic guidance using the 3.2 drill followed by tapping. Compression slot screw was used at the end to compress the fracture under fluoroscopy control.

The wound was then copiously irrigated. The IT band was closed with 0 Vicryl. The subcutaneous layer was closed with a running 2-0 Vicryl stitch. The skin was closed with staples. A medium Hemovac was placed in the deep layer of closure before the wound was actually closed. The patient was extubated and transferred to the recovery room in stable conditions.

Attending staff was present during the whole procedure.

Chapter 32

Percutaneous Sacroiliac Joint Screw Fixation

Karim Masrouha, M.D.

COMMON INDICATIONS

- Unstable posterior pelvic ring fractures (AP3, LC3, Vertical shear)
- Sacroiliac joint dislocations
- Sacral fractures
- Anatomic reduction achievable through closed or open techniques

CONTRAINDICATIONS

- Sacral dysmorphism (relative)
- Obesity (relative)
- Inability to achieve a closed anatomic reduction
- Severely comminuted sacral fracture
- Inability to obtain excellent fluoroscopic visualization

POSSIBLE COMPLICATIONS

- Screw misplacement
- Fixation failure
- Delayed union
- Nonunion
- Deep pelvic infection
- S1 nerve root injury (inferior and posterior)
- L5 nerve root injury (superior and anterior)

S. Saghieh et al. (eds.), *Operative Dictations in Orthopedic Surgery*,
DOI 10.1007/978-1-4614-7479-1_32,
© Springer Science+Business Media New York 2013

ESSENTIAL STEPS
1. Supine positioning
2. Bolster under the sacrum and lumbar spine
3. Evaluation of fluoroscopic images to confirm ability to safely place screws percutaneously
4. Reduction of pelvis
5. Obtain perfect inlet, outlet, and lateral views
6. Mark radiographic landmarks based off the lateral image
7. Stab incision
8. Orientation of guide wire with the use of modified cannulated guide
9. Placement of screw under fluoroscopic control
10. Evaluation of reduction and hardware prior to leaving the operating room out of traction

OPERATIVE NOTE
Indications: ____-year-old male/female with sacroiliac joint dislocation/sacral fracture/posterior pelvic fracture

Preoperative Diagnosis: Sacroiliac joint dislocation/sacral fracture/posterior pelvic fracture

Procedure: Percutaneous sacroiliac joint screw fixation

Postoperative Diagnosis: Same

Description of Operation: The patient and surgical site were identified and marked. We confirmed that a bowel prep had been completed the night prior to surgery. The patient then underwent anesthesia per the anesthesia team. The patient was positioned in the supine position on a fluoroscopically compatible operating table. Intravenous antibiotics were administered.

The patient was elevated from the table and a folded blanket was placed under the lumbosacral spine to elevate the pelvis off the table. The C-arm was positioned to come into the field from the left side. An antero-posterior view of the pelvis was obtained to center the pubic symphysis over the center of the sacrum. An inlet view of the pelvis was then obtained by tilting the image intensifier until the anterior cortical ring of S1 and S2 were superimposed as concentric circles. The position of the C-arm was then recorded. An outlet view was then obtained by tilting the C-arm 90° caudal and visualizing the superior aspect of the pubic symphysis over the S2 vertebral body. The position of the C-arm was then recorded.

A distal transfemoral traction pin was placed from the medial to lateral side taking care to prevent injury to the medial neurovascular structures. The right/left leg was placed in 25 lb of traction. The anterior pelvic fixator that had been in place the day of injury (1 day prior) was loosened slightly while the longitudinal traction was applied through the right/left lower extremity. Lateral compression was maintained manually and the fixator was secured. Repeat imaging following the reduction maneuvers showed an anatomic reduction on both pelvis views. The C-arm position for the perfect inlet and outlet views was reconfirmed.

The flanks, pelvis, groin, and bilateral lower extremities were prepped with betadine/chlorhexidine. The operative site was toweled off (including the groin) and secured with skin staples. An impervious U-drape was placed over the abdomen with the tails extending distally. A second U-drape was placed under the pelvis extending proximally. The right lower extremity was circumferentially prepped out below the level of the traction pin. The C-arm was brought in and rotated to a lateral view. A true lateral view was obtained by superimposing the greater sciatic notches. A free guide wire was then used to mark the anterior border of the sacrum, posterior border of the sacrum, superior endplate of S1, and the projection of the sacral ala. These skin markings allowed us to see the location of our entry point distal to the alar line between the anterior and posterior borders of the sacrum. The orientation was marked on the skin for superior, inferior, anterior, and posterior relative to the sacrum and therefore the orthogonal pelvic images. A 1 cm longitudinal incision was then made over the posterosuperior aspect of the window and spread down to the lateral ilium. A modified cannulated guide was then inserted onto the lateral ilium and the position relative to the window for the S1 foramen was checked radiographically. An extra long threaded tip guide wire was then placed through the cannulated guide and the outlet view was evaluated for the wire position in the superior–inferior orientation. Minor adjustments were made and the wire was then evaluated with the inlet view for the AP orientation. After confirming proper alignment, the guide wire was advanced directed into the body of the S1. When the wire was in the area of the foramen, both the outlet and inlet views were evaluated to confirm proper position. The length of the wire was measured and the path was drilled over the wire. A self-tapping 105 mm partially threaded 7.3 mm cannulated screw was then placed with a washer to provide compression across the SI joint. Orthogonal views confirmed proper positioning. A second stab incision was then made over the anteroinferior aspect of the window. A second parallel screw was placed through the window in a similar fashion as above.

The wounds were irrigated with normal saline and closed with skin staples. The external fixator junctions were checked to ensure security. Plain film inlet and outlet views were obtained without traction. The wounds were dressed. After confirming maintenance of reduction and adequate hardware placement, the patient was awakened from general anesthesia and transferred to recovery in good condition. No intra-operative complications.

Staff was present and scrubbed for the entire procedure.

Chapter 33

Supracondylar Femur Open Reduction and Internal Fixation

Moustapha Awada, M.D.

INDICATIONS
- Extraarticular supracondylar femur fracture
- Some simple intraarticular supracondylar femur fracture
- Some distal femur shaft fracture

POSSIBLE COMPLICATIONS
- Malunion with axial deviation in sagittal or frontal plane
- Nonunion
- Failure of the fixation
- DVT/Pulmonary embolism
- Fat embolism
- Superficial or deep infection

ESSENTIAL STEPS
1. Positioning
2. Reduction under fluoroscopy
3. Placement of guide pin
4. Reaming of femoral canal
5. Placement of nail
6. Placement of proximal and distal locking screws

OPERATIVE NOTE
Indications: Patient is a ___- year-old M/F who was hit by a car. He/she was transferred to the emergency room where he/she was diagnosed with an isolated left/right closed supracondylar femur fracture with extension to the articular surface.

S. Saghieh et al. (eds.), *Operative Dictations in Orthopedic Surgery*,
DOI 10.1007/978-1-4614-7479-1_33,
© Springer Science+Business Media New York 2013

Preoperative Diagnosis: Closed right/left supracondylar femur fracture

Procedure: Retrograde intramedullary nailing of right/left supracondylar femur fracture

Postoperative Diagnosis: Same

Description of Operation: The patient was identified in the preoperative holding area and brought to the operating room. He/she was placed supine on the operating table. General endotracheal anesthesia was administered and IV antibiotics given.

A bump was placed under the right/left hip and all pressure points were well padded. The left/right lower extremity was then prepped and draped in the usual sterile fashion.

The knee was bent over a bolster and closed reduction attempted under fluoroscopy. A small 1-cm incision was made on the medial and lateral femoral condyles to insert a large reduction tenaculum clamp to help in achieving and maintaining reduction of the articular surface. Two guide pins were used to fix the intercondylar extension of the fracture. They were parallel to the articular surface and posterior to the intramedullary nail tract. Two 7 mm cannulated screws were inserted over the guide pins after appropriate drilling and tapping.

A 6 cm longitudinal incision was made over the patellar tendon region. The subcutaneous tissues were dissected with tissue scissors to the level of the patellar tendon.

The patellar tendon was incised longitudinally throughout its length. Fluoroscopy was used to place a guide pin in the intercondylar notch near the region of the most anterior aspect of Blumensaat's line. The drill was then used to advance the guide pin into the femoral canal across the fracture fragment while maintaining anatomic reduction with manual traction. The 10 mm drill bit was then used to ream over the guide pin maintaining anatomic alignment. The femoral canal was then reamed to xx mm by 1-mm increments using fluoroscopy. Sizing of the nail was performed and the appropriate nail was then introduced under fluoroscopic guidance. The fracture was held in anatomic alignment during nail placement. The distal locking screws were then placed under fluoroscopy using the guide apparatus. They measured xx mm, xx mm, and xx mm in length. The two proximal interlocking screws were then placed using the guide apparatus as well. These measured xx mm in length. Final alignment of the nail and the internal components was reassessed and found to be acceptable under fluoroscopic evaluation. The wounds were then irrigated with sterile saline. The patellar tendon was closed with a running 0 Vicryl suture. The paratenon was closed with an undyed

2-0 Vicryl suture. The subcutaneous tissues of all incisions were closed with 2-0 Vicryl. The skin at all incisions was closed with interrupted 3-0 nylon sutures. A sterile dressing was applied followed by Ace wrap. The knee was placed in an immobilizer. The patient tolerated the procedure well. He/she was extubated in the operating room and transported to the recovery room in stable condition. Blood loss estimation was ___ cc. Attending staff was present and scrubbed for the entire procedure.

Chapter 34

Bipolar Hemiarthroplasty

Said Saghieh, M.D.

COMMON INDICATIONS
- Displaced femoral neck fracture

POSSIBLE COMPLICATIONS
- Risks of anesthesia
- Infection
- Thromboembolic phenomenon
- Neurocirculatory compromise
- Hip dislocation
- Stiffness
- Hip or thigh pain
- Leg length inequality
- Late loosening

ESSENTIAL STEPS
1. Positioning
2. Posterior approach
3. Osteotomy of the femoral neck
4. Extraction of femoral head
5. Preparation of the femoral canal
6. Insertion of the prosthesis
7. Reduction
8. Closure

OPERATIVE NOTE
Preoperative Diagnosis: Displaced femoral neck fracture
Procedure: Bipolar hemiarthroplasty

S. Saghieh et al. (eds.), *Operative Dictations in Orthopedic Surgery*,
DOI 10.1007/978-1-4614-7479-1_34,
© Springer Science+Business Media New York 2013

Postoperative Diagnosis: Same

Indication: This is a ____year-old M/F who fell down 12 hours before and sustained a displaced fracture of the R/L femoral neck.

Description of Operation: After induction of general anesthesia, prophylactic antibiotics were given. A Foley catheter was applied. The patient was placed in the lateral decubitus position over a bean bag. All bony prominences were well padded. The lower extremity was prepped and draped for surgery. Skin incision started at the posterior 1/3 of the greater trochanter and extended proximally for 8 cm toward a point 2 fingerbreadths below the PSIS. The incision was then extended distally over the lateral side of the thigh for 5 cm. The incision was carried through the subcutaneous tissue and iliotibial band. The Charnley bow was placed. The posterior aspect of the hip was addressed first, placing a Hohmann between capsule and gluteus minimus. The piriformis, conjoint tendon, obturator externus, and quadratus femoris were incised off their insertion into the greater trochanter. The fracture was identified. The femoral neck was cut one finger breadth proximal to the lesser trochanter according to the template. The femoral head was retrieved with the corkscrew tool and measured. The labrum was excised. The femur was flexed and internally rotated to 90°. A jaws retractor was placed anteriorly, a curved cobra was placed medially, and a bent Hohmann was placed laterally. The residual external rotators were removed. A cookie cutter followed by a T-bar reamer and pilot hole reamer were used. The femoral canal was sequentially reamed to the appropriate diameter as planned. The broach was placed anatomically in approximately 10–15° of anteversion. The calcar was reamed. The appropriately sized ball was placed on the neck. The hip was located. Range of motion was measured and found to be acceptable. The leg length appeared equal. All the trial components were removed. Pulse lavage was performed. The femoral component was inserted with appropriate press fit and anteversion. The appropriate ball was placed onto the femoral head and relocated into the acetabulum being sure as to have no soft tissue interposition. The external rotators and capsules were reapproximated to the greater trochanter through drill holes. A drain was placed deep to the IT band coming through the anterolateral skin. #1 running PDS was used for IT band closure. #1 PDS in two layers was used for subcutaneous closure. 2-0 Prolene interrupted vertical mattress, staples, Adaptic, fluffs, and bias stockinette were applied. The patient was placed supine, placed on the hospital bed, and taken to the recovery room in satisfactory condition.

There were no immediate complications noted.

A Staff member was present and scrubbed for the entire procedure.

Chapter 35
Iliac Crest Bone Graft (Anterior)

Said Saghieh, M.D.

COMMON INDICATIONS

- To fill cavities or defects resulting from curettage of benign tumors.
- To bridge defects of a long bone or in a joint (arthrodesis).
- To promote union in fresh fractures, or after osteotomies.
- To treat delayed union and nonunion.

POSSIBLE COMPLICATIONS

- Hernias.
- Lateral femoral cutaneous and ilioinguinal nerves are at risk during harvest of bone from the anterior ilium.
- Cosmetic deformity if large amount of bone removed.
- Pain at site of harvest.
- Bleeding.
- Fracture of iliac bone.

ESSENTIAL STEPS

1. Skin incision
2. Fascia incision and dissection of the abdominal muscles off the iliac crest
3. Cortical bone window
4. Harvest medullary cavity with gouges, curettes
5. Closure

S. Saghieh et al. (eds.), *Operative Dictations in Orthopedic Surgery*,
DOI 10.1007/978-1-4614-7479-1_35,
© Springer Science+Business Media New York 2013

OPERATIVE NOTE

Indications: History: this is a ___-year-old M/F who has a delayed union of the tibia fracture. Autogenous iliac bone graft was advised.

Preoperative Diagnosis: Delayed Union of tibia fracture

Procedure: Autogeneous Iliac crest bone grafting (r/l)

Postoperative Diagnosis: Same

Description of Operation: The patient was identified and side marked in the preoperative holding area. He/she was brought into the operative suite and placed supine on the operating table. IV antibiotics were given. General endotracheal anesthesia was induced without difficulty. The R/L anterior flank was prepped and draped in the usual sterile manner. An oblique 3 cm skin incision was made parallel and slightly inferior to the iliac crest. The incision started 2.5 cm posterior to the anterosuperior iliac spine. It was deepened through the subcutaneous tissue. The fascia was incised. The abdominal muscles were reflected off the iliac crest. Subperiosteal dissection was done on the outer table of the ilium and a Taylor retractor was used to retract the muscles off. With a straight half inch osteotome, a 1.5 cm length cortical window was designed. A curve osteotome was used to complete the window taking into consideration to spare the inner cortex. Straight and curve curettes and gouges were used through the cortical window to harvest cancellous bone without breaking through the inner and the outer tables.

Once the procedure was completed, this wound was irrigated with copious amounts of saline and closed in anatomical layers; the fascia with vicryl 0, the subcutaneous with vicryl 2.0, and the skin with subcuticular 3-0 Monocryl.

A sterile dressing was applied.

Part IV
Knee and Leg

Chapter 36

Primary Total Knee Arthroplasty

Said Saghieh, M.D.

COMMON INDICATIONS

- Primary or secondary osteoarthritis of the knee
- Rheumatoid arthritis
- Arthropathy secondary to hemophilia
- Malalignment producing asymmetric wearing of the knee
- All leading to significant impairment of ambulation and failing to respond to more conservative treatment

POSSIBLE COMPLICATIONS

- Infection
- Thromboembolic phenomenon
- Neurocirculatory compromise
- dislocation
- Stiffness
- Patella maltracking
- Patella fracture
- Patellar tendon rupture
- Late loosening

ESSENTIAL STEPS

1. Templating of radiographs
2. Incision of skin and soft tissues
3. Medial arthrotomy
4. Eversion of the patella
5. Cut the cruciate ligaments and menisci
6. Release of the MCL
7. Distal femoral cut
8. Tibial cut
9. Extension gap measurement

S. Saghieh et al. (eds.), *Operative Dictations in Orthopedic Surgery*,
DOI 10.1007/978-1-4614-7479-1_36,
© Springer Science+Business Media New York 2013

10. Sizing the femur and the four in one femoral cuts
11. Flexion gap measurement
12. Final tibia preparation
13. Placement of trial components
14. Placement of permanent components
15. Closure

OPERATIVE NOTE

Preoperative Diagnosis: Knee osteoarthritis, L/R
Procedure: Cemented total knee replacement, L/R
Postoperative Diagnosis: Same
Indication: The patient is a ___-year-old male/female with severe knee pain and difficulty with ambulation secondary to osteoarthritis. He/she failed conservative treatment including intraarticular steroid injection.
Description of Operation:
Implants Used:

> Company
> Femoral component
> Tibia component
> Polyethylene

The patient was identified in the holding area and the affected extremity marked. He/she was brought into the operating room and placed in a supine position. General endotracheal anesthesia was preformed by the anesthesia team. The patient was given prophylactic antibiotics, a Foley was inserted, and the tourniquet applied over the proximal thigh. All bony prominences were well padded. The ____ leg was prepped and draped for surgery. The tourniquet was inflated to ____ mmHg. A midline incision was carried out starting 6 cm proximal to the patella, going over the patella and distally 1 cm medial to the tibial tubercle. The incision was carried through the subcutaneous tissue. The quadriceps tendon was identified and incised longitudinally on its medial portion. The dissection proceeded distally with a medial parapatellar arthrotomy. The anterior fad pad was excised and the patellar tendon was released off the bone for few mm to allow tension-free lateral eversion of the patella. The medial and lateral menisci, the anterior cruciate ligament and the proximal part of the posterior cruciate ligament were excised. The medial collateral ligament was released from the tibial plateau to the posteromedial corner.

With the knee bent 90°, the femur intramedullary jig was inserted with ___ degrees of valgus as preplanned on preoperative radiographs. The distal femoral cut was done. Then the intramedullary tibia jig was inserted and the proximal tibia cut was performed perpendicular to the tibia axis. Extension gap was assessed. There was good mediolateral symmetry, with 10 mm extension block fitting well. There was no flexion contracture. The knee was brought again into flexion. The distal femur was sized and the appropriate 4-x-1 jig applied in 3° of external rotation to match the epicondylar axis. The bone cuts and the chamfer cuts were made. Flexion gap was assessed. It was symmetrical and matched the extension gap thickness. The intercondylar box jig was applied next and the intercondylar box was prepared.

The patella was measured to be ___ mm. It was osteotomized to ___ mm. Three drill holes were placed in the patella. The appropriate patellar trial component was placed.

The femoral and tibial trial components were placed. A final alignment test was performed. The rotation for the tibia tray was set. The patella tracking was assessed.

The femoral, the patellar components, and the plastic tibia spacer were removed. The final tibial preparation was performed with the intramedullary central drill followed by the punch and its flanges.

After thorough irrigation, the bone surfaces were dried and the final femur, tibia, and patellar components were cemented in. The appropriate size trial articular spacer was used and the knee was brought into neutral extension to allow the settling of the cement. A clamp was used to hold the patellar button in place. The excess of cement was removed from around the tibia and femur.

After the cement has set, the appropriate polyethylene spacer was inserted. The tourniquet was let down for a total tourniquet time of _____. Hemostasis was achieved with electrocautery. A hemovac drain was placed deep to the quadriceps mechanism coming through the anterolateral skin. The extensor mechanism was closed with #1 Vicryl. The subcutaneous tissues were closed with 2-0 Vicryl. The skin was closed with staplers. Adaptic, fluffs, and Jones dressing were applied. The patient was awakened, placed on the hospital bed, and taken to the recovery room in satisfactory condition.

There were no intraoperative complications.

Faculty was present for the entire procedure.

Postoperative rehabilitation: Early range of motion using a continuous passive motion machine. Extension should be achieved early and flexion should be at 90° by the time of discharge from the hospital. Patient is full-weight bearing on the first postoperative day and use a walker/cane until sufficient quadriceps strength has returned.

Chapter 37
Medial Unicompartmental Knee Replacement

Said Saghieh, M.D.

COMMON INDICATIONS
- Left/right knee isolated medial compartment arthritis
- Intact cruciate ligaments

CONTRAINDICATIONS
- Very obese patient
- Patella baha
- Previous high tibial osteotomy

POSSIBLE COMPLICATIONS
- Infection
- Thromboembolic phenomenon
- Neurocirculatory compromise
- Fracture dislocation
- Stiffness
- Patellar problems
- Late loosening

ESSENTIAL STEPS
1. Incision
2. Tibia jig and cut
3. Femoral jig and cut
4. Closure

S. Saghieh et al. (eds.), *Operative Dictations in Orthopedic Surgery*,
DOI 10.1007/978-1-4614-7479-1_37,
© Springer Science+Business Media New York 2013

OPERATIVE NOTE

Indications: This is a ___-year-old F/M who has been complaining of R/L knee pain over the past 3 years. The pain is not controlled by NSAID and intraarticular injections. Radiographs revealed an isolated medial compartment arthritis. There is a mild varus deformity and no clinical signs of cruciate ligament tear.

Preoperative Diagnosis: R/L knee medial compartment arthritis

Procedure: Cemented unicondylar knee replacement

Postoperative Diagnosis: Same

Description of Operation: Implants Used:

The patient was identified in the holding area and the affected extremity marked. He/she was brought into the operating room and placed in a supine position. General endotracheal anesthesia was performed by the anesthesia team. The patient was given prophylactic antibiotics, a Foley was inserted, and the tourniquet applied. All extremities were well padded. The ____ leg was prepped and draped for surgery. The tourniquet was inflated to 350 mmHg.

A 10 cm longitudinal skin incision was carried out over the right/left knee just medial to the midline of the patella starting at the superior pole of the patella going distally 2–3 cm distal to the joint line. A medial parapatellar arthrotomy was then performed. The anterior fat pad was excised as well as the medial meniscus. The patient had intact anterior cruciate and posterior cruciate ligaments. Periosteum was elevated from the medial side of the proximal tibia along the joint line back towards, but not into, the collateral ligament. Subperiosteal dissection was carried laterally as well to reach the patellar tendon insertion. The medial osteophytes were removed off from the medial tibial plateau and the medial femoral condyle. With an electrocautery, a line was drawn medial to the ACL tibial insertion. The proximal tibial cutting jig was assembled and fixed to the bone. Sagittal and frontal alignment were checked. A reciprocating blade was used at the base of the tibial eminence to cut, along the edge of the ACL down to, but not beyond, the intended level of the transverse cut. The transverse bone cut was fashioned to remove approximately 4 mm of tibial plateau with 1.27 mm oscillating saw blade introduced through the slot in the cutting guide. A retractor was used medially to protect the medial collateral ligament. The tibia jig was removed.

Flexion and extension gaps were checked to be satisfactory.

The cartilage of the distal femoral condyle was shaved with a saw. The femoral jig was applied and checked to be parallel to the tibia cut.

The femoral cut was performed with 1.27 mm oscillating saw blade introduced through the slot in the cutting guide.

The femur was sized, the appropriate chamfer and posterior cuts were made. The jig was removed and gaps again checked.

The tibial plate was sized. The appropriate pegs were drilled.

A femoral trial was placed followed by the tibial trial and 10 mm insert. The patient went from full extension to 125° of flexion. Cement was pressurized onto the femur. The femoral component was applied. Residual cement was removed. Cement was pressurized onto the tibia. The components were brought out to full extension. After doing this, we tried our best to get out all the posterior cement around the femur and the tibia. The 10 mm insert was placed. The knee was brought into extension. The tourniquet was let down. Bleeders were cauterized. The retinaculum was closed with #1 PDS. 2-0 Vicryl was used for subcutaneous closure after placing a deep drain. Staples were used for skin. Adaptic and fluffs were applied. The patient was awakened and taken to the Recovery Room in satisfactory condition.

There were no intraoperative complications.

Faculty was present for the entire procedure.

Chapter 38

Distal Femoral Varus Osteotomy

Said Saghieh, M.D.

COMMON INDICATIONS
- Genu valgum with mechanical axis of the lower extremity passing lateral to the knee joint center and lateral distal femoral angle less than 85°.

POSSIBLE COMPLICATIONS
- Under- or over-correction
- Loss of fixation
- Infection
- Knee stiffness
- DVT

ESSENTIAL STEPS
1. Patient position on OR table
2. Lateral skin incision
3. Guide wire placement under fluoroscopy
4. Osteotomy at correct sagittal and coronal angle
5. Open osteotomy without fracturing medial cortex
6. Apply puddu plate, graft
7. Closure

OPERATIVE NOTE
This is a ___-year-old patient who has genu valgum deformity and early lateral compartment arthritis. Scanogram showed a valgus distal femur with a lateral distal femoral angle of ___. The medial proximal tibia angle was within normal values. The pros and cons of surgery were explained to the patient.

S. Saghieh et al. (eds.), *Operative Dictations in Orthopedic Surgery*,
DOI 10.1007/978-1-4614-7479-1_38,
© Springer Science+Business Media New York 2013

Preoperative Diagnosis: R/L knee joint valgus deformity with early lateral unicompartmental degeneration

Procedure: Distal femur varus osteotomy with puddu plate with application of tricalcium hydroxyapatite bone graft substitute

Postoperative Diagnosis: Same

Description of Operation: The patient was identified in the preoperative holding area and the involved extremity was marked. The patient was brought into the operative suite and placed supine on the operating table. General endotracheal anesthesia was induced and prophylactic IV antibiotics were given. A tourniquet was placed over soft-roll on the proximal thigh. The operated limb including the ipsilateral hip was prepped free, and a small bump was placed under the hip. The preoperative drawings were reviewed showing for a desired correction of $x°$, the opening wedge would have to be xx mm at the femur osteotomy site.

A 10-cm skin incision was made over the lateral aspect of the distal femur, starting distally at the Gerdy's tubercle. The iliotibial band was incised in line with the incision, and the vastus lateralis was then dissected posteriorly off the lateral intermuscular septum. Subperiosteal dissection was carried out with Cobb elevator to expose the femur from the insertion of the joint capsule to a point sufficiently proximal to accommodate the side plate. With the use of fluoroscopy, the starting point for the osteotomy was located 3 cm above the lateral femoral epicondyle. A guide pin was introduced from that point and directed distally and medially to exit the cortex at the level of the medial epicondyle. It was angled about 10–15° from anterior to posterior to keep it centered within the condyles. A second guide pin was inserted parallel and posterior to the first one.

The osteotomy was then performed with a 1-in. oscillating saw using both pins as a guide. Wide osteotomes were used to complete the osteotomy leaving the medial cortex intact to act as a hinge. Successively larger size wedged osteotomes were utilized to continue the wedging process. Then a distraction device is placed in the osteotomy site and slowly distracted to open the osteotomy to the predetermined width of xx mm as determined by the preoperative long standing view x-rays.

Once this had been in place, the appropriate plate was inserted into the opened osteotomy site and tamped into place. ___ proximal and ___ distal screws were used for plate fixation.

Fluoroscopy was utilized to check position of the screws. Wedge bone graft substitute was used to fill the defect.

The tourniquet was deflated. The wound was thoroughly irrigated and hemostasis achieved. The wound was closed in three layers; the fascia with 0 Vicryl in a figure-of-eight interrupted fashion, the subcutaneous tissue with 2-0 Vicryl in a running fashion, and the skin with 3-0 Monocryl in a subcuticular fashion. Sterile dressings were applied. The patient was placed in a knee immobilizer and then was awakened and taken out of the operative suite to the post-op recovery room in excellent condition without any evidence of immediate complications.

Staff was present and scrubbed during the whole procedure.

Chapter 39
High Tibial Osteotomy (Closing Wedge)

Karim Masrouha, M.D.

COMMON INDICATIONS
- Medial compartment knee osteoarthritis

POSSIBLE COMPLICATIONS
- Infection
- Thromboembolism
- Fractures
- Compartment syndrome
- Delayed union/nonunion
- Neurovascular injury
- Under correction

ESSENTIAL STEPS
1. Preoperative assessment and planning (history, physical examination, evaluation of radiographs)
2. Protection of the patellar tendon anteriorly and the neurovascular structure posteriorly
3. Care must be taken to cut through to the posterolateral corner and medially so that the tibia has "greenstick" looseness
4. The osteotomy is compressed with a compression clamp and secured by tightening the screws
5. Irrigation and incision closure
6. Long-leg cast application and strict elevation

S. Saghieh et al. (eds.), *Operative Dictations in Orthopedic Surgery*,
DOI 10.1007/978-1-4614-7479-1_39,
© Springer Science+Business Media New York 2013

OPERATIVE NOTE

Preoperative Diagnosis: Medial compartment osteoarthritis/tibia vara
Procedure: High tibial osteotomy (closing wedge)
Postoperative Diagnosis: Same
Indications: ____ -year-old male/female with tibia vara developed medial compartment osteoarthritis
Description of Operation: The patient and surgical site were identified and marked. The patient then underwent anesthesia per the anesthesia team. The patient was positioned in the supine position on the operative table with a hip bump in addition to a foot bump to keep the knee in hyperflexion. The limb was scrubbed and draped in the standard sterile fashion. A tourniquet was placed on the thigh over a soft-roll. Intravenous antibiotics were administered.

An inverted L-shaped incision was made just below the level of the joint line that extends posteriorly just past the fibular head, anteriorly to the patellar tendon, and inferiorly along the lateral side of the tibia for 10 cm. The incision was deepened through the patellar paratenon and bluntly spread. A retractor was used to protect the patellar tendon. The incision was then carried down to the periosteum and the anterior compartment muscles were elevated off the cortical surface. The tibio-fibular joint was then disrupted with an osteotome and the fibula was then displaced posteriorly. A retractor was then passed posterior to the tibia to protect the neurovascular and posterior muscles.

On each of the medial and lateral sides of the tibia, two Keith needles were inserted into the proximal tibial joint line from front to back. A transverse osteotomy guide was placed, positioning the jig 2 cm beneath the joint line and tightened. A pin was then inserted in the posterior jig hole and a plate applied over it, ensuring that it was parallel to the joint line. A second pin was then inserted for stabilization. The tibial width was measured with a depth gauge after drilling through the central hole.

After inserting retractors to protect the posterior neurovascular structures and the patellar tendon the tibia was cut with a saw 2 cm beneath the joint line from the lateral aspect to the medial, including the posterolateral corner, leaving 1 cm of the medial tibia.

The oblique osteotomy jig was then applied over the guide pins and a cut was made so that the saw blade intersected with the previous cut and the wedge was removed.

An L-shaped plate was then applied over the smooth pins which were then replaced with 6.5 mm cortical screws that were inserted loosely. A 3.2 mm hole through one cortex was made in line with the distal plate and a compression clamp was placed through it to compress the osteotomy. The plate was then secured by tightening the cortical screws. Incisions were irrigated and closed with 2-vicryl and 3-0 nylon or PDS.

No intra-operative complications.

Staff was present and scrubbed for entire procedure.

Postoperative regimen: Application of a long-leg cast. Strict elevation of the knee above the heart for 5 days. Non-weight bearing for 8 weeks followed by progressive weight bearing over 4 weeks with physical therapy and muscle strengthening exercises.

Chapter 40
Medial Opening Wedge Tibial Osteotomy

Said Saghieh, M.D.

COMMON INDICATIONS
- Isolated medial compartment osteoarthritis

CONTRAINDICATIONS
- Patella baha
- Lateral instability/subluxation
- Limited range of motion
- Advanced age
- Obesity
- Lateral compartment OA
- Medial compartment depression

POSSIBLE COMPLICATIONS
- Recurrence of deformity
- Infection
- Fracture
- Nonunion
- Patella baha

ESSENTIAL STEPS
1. Preoperative planning to determine size of opening wedge
2. Subperiosteal dissection to expose proximal surface of tibia

S. Saghieh et al. (eds.), *Operative Dictations in Orthopedic Surgery*,
DOI 10.1007/978-1-4614-7479-1_40,
© Springer Science+Business Media New York 2013

3. Cortical cut with saw and completion of osteotomy
4. Opening of wedge to planned size
5. Fixation of opening with plate
6. Bone graft of wedge space
7. Closure

OPERATIVE NOTE

Preoperative Diagnosis: Medial compartment osteoarthritis, L/R knee

Procedure Medial Opening wedge high tibial osteotomy

Postoperative Diagnosis: Same

Indications: The patient is a _____year-old F/M who has medial compartment osteoarthritis and good lateral joint space who has failed conservative treatment of his/her knee pain. The patient was thus indicated for a high tibial osteotomy to decrease pressure on the medial compartment. The patient, after discussion of the risks and benefits of the procedure, wishes to proceed with high tibial osteotomy. Long leg standing x-rays of the lower extremity were evaluated and templated for operative planning to address the amount of correction desired.

Description of Operation: The patient was identified in the preoperative holding area and the involved extremity was marked. The patient was brought to the operating room and positioned supine on the operating table. General (or regional) anesthesia was induced by the anesthesiologist. All pressure points were well padded. Pre-op IV antibiotics (name and dose) were administered. A thigh tourniquet was placed, and the extremity was prepped and draped in a sterile fashion. Elastic bandage was used to exsanguinate the limb, and the tourniquet was inflated to _____ mm Hg. A 7 cm longitudinal skin incision was made approximately 3 cm medial to the tibial tubercle, and blunt dissection was used to reach the level of the pes anserinus tendons. These were elevated and retracted posteriorly along with the superficial medial collateral ligament.

Subperiosteal dissection was performed to expose borders of the bone A retractor was placed posteriorly to protect the MCL and neurovascular structures. Anteriorly, a retractor was used to protect the patellar tendon.

Under fluoroscopic image intensification, two parallel 2.5-mm guidewires were placed in the subchondral bone parallel to the joint line.

The appropriate jig was applied and Two K-wires were inserted along the plane of the osteotomy going obliquely from distal medial to proximal lateral toward the tibiofibular joint. A sagittal saw was placed distal to the guidewires and was passed parallel to the K-wires approximately two-thirds of the way across the tibia avoiding penetrating the lateral cortex.

An osteotome was then used to separate the anterior and posterior cortices and was advanced laterally within 1 cm of the lateral cortex.

A gradual distraction instrument was introduced into the osteotomy site to assist with achieving the appropriate amount of correction as determined by the preoperative planning.

The corresponding plate was applied to the tibia with two distal and two proximal screws to fix the osteotomy in the open position.

Tourniquet was deflated, and the total tourniquet time was ____. Hemostasis was achieved. The wound was irrigated.

The opening was packed with a wedge of bone graft (___). The pes anserinus was closed over the plate with vicryl 0, the subcutaneous tissue was closed with vicryl 2.0, and the skin was closed with monocryl 4.0 in subcuticular fashion. A sterile dressing was applied. The patient was awakened from anesthesia and was transported to the recovery room in satisfactory condition. There were no immediate complications associated with the procedure.

A staff was present and scrubbed through the entire procedure.

Chapter 41

Arthroscopic Meniscectomy of the Knee

Hamdi G. Sukkarieh, M.D.

COMMON INDICATIONS
- Unstable, irreparable tears of the meniscus that are sufficiently symptomatic

CONTRAINDICATIONS
- Significant osteoarthritis of the knee

POSSIBLE COMPLICATIONS
- Nerve or blood vessel damage
- Bleeding and hemarthrosis
- Infection
- Stiffening of the knee joint
- Failure of the procedure
- Thromboembolic disease
- Anesthetic complications
- Instrument failure
- Reflex sympathetic dystrophy
- Ligament injury
- Fracture
- Iatrogenic injuries to articular surfaces

ESSENTIAL STEPS
1. Position patient supine
2. Apply tourniquet to upper thigh
3. Distend joint by injecting 60 cm³ NS

S. Saghieh et al. (eds.), *Operative Dictations in Orthopedic Surgery*,
DOI 10.1007/978-1-4614-7479-1_41,
© Springer Science+Business Media New York 2013

4. Select portal sites and insert scope
5. Perform a complete arthroscopic examination of the knee
6. Thoroughly probe torn meniscus to accurately determine the type of tear
7. Remove torn/mobile fragment and contour remaining peripheral rim

OPERATIVE NOTE

Preoperative Diagnosis: Right/Left knee medial/lateral irrepairable symptomatic meniscal tear

Procedure: Arthroscopic medial/lateral meniscectomy, right/left knee

Postoperative Diagnosis: Same

Indications: This is a ___-year-old M/F who has been complaining of R/L knee pain, mild swelling and locking events for the past 3 months. MRI revealed a tear of the medial/lateral meniscus.

Description of Operation:

The patient was brought to the operating room and placed supine on the operating table. After adequate anesthesia was provided, the nonoperative extremity was placed in the well-leg holder. A tourniquet was placed on the thigh of the operative extremity. All pressure points were padded. The patient was then prepped and draped in the standard surgical fashion.

With an Esmarch bandage, the lower extremity was exsanguinated and the tourniquet was inflated to 250 mmHg. An 18-gauge spinal needle was placed into the joint and 60 cm^3 of NS was injected. An 11 blade was used to make a 1 cm long skin incision located 1 cm above the joint line and 1 cm medial to the patellar tendon. The incision was deepened through the joint capsule. The arthroscope was introduced into the joint. A similar incision was made 1 cm lateral to the patellar tendon. Under direct visualization via the arthroscope, the incision was deepened through the joint capsule. Diagnostic arthroscopy began with examination of the medial compartment. The articular surface of the tibia demonstrated (grade ___ chondromalacia). No loose bodies or osteophytes were seen. The medial meniscus was found to have a ___ cm radial oblique tear extending posteriorly. The torn portion was mobile. The remainder of the meniscus was intact and secure.

Examination of the intercondylar notch revealed that the ACL and PCL were completely intact. No loose bodies or osteophytes were seen. The arthroscope was moved to the lateral compartment. The articular surfaces of the femur and tibia were normal.

The lateral meniscus was intact. No loose bodies or osteophytes were seen. Examination continued into the lateral gutter. No loose bodies or osteophytes were seen. The synovium appeared normal. The patellofemoral joint was examined and found to have normal articular surfaces. No osteophytes or loose bodies were seen. The suprapatellar pouch was also free of loose bodies and the synovium appeared normal. The arthroscope was moved into the medial gutter. No osteophytes or loose bodies were seen. The synovium appeared normal. Attention returned to the medial compartment. Using the arthroscopic instruments (biters, graspers, coblaters, shavers), the torn portion of the medial meniscus was grasped and amputated at its base. The motorized shaver was then used to contour the remaining portion of the meniscus. The instruments were removed and the tourniquet deflated. The portals were closed with 3-0 nylon suture placed in a simple fashion. A clean dressing was applied. Staff was present and scrubbed during the procedure.

Postoperative Rehabilitation

Following arthroscopic meniscectomy, patients are routinely able to

- walk without support within 1–3 days
- return to work after 1–2 weeks
- resume athletic training by 2–4 weeks
- return to competition in 3–4 weeks

Physiotherapy has not always shown benefit except in cases of preoperative deficits.

Chapter 42
ACL Reconstruction

Brian R. Wolf, M.D., M.S.

COMMON INDICATIONS
- Knee instability from anterior cruciate ligament (ACL) deficiency

POSSIBLE COMPLICATIONS
- Patella fracture
- Graft fracture
- Patellar or quadriceps tendon avulsions
- Graft failure or rerupture
- Motion loss
- Patellofemoral symptoms

ESSENTIAL STEPS
1. Diagnostic knee arthroscopy and debridement of torn ACL
2. Graft harvest
3. Notchplasty if needed
4. Identification of tibial ACL footprint and placement of tibial tunnel
5. Identification of femoral footprint and drilling of femoral tunnel
6. Graft passage, tensioning, and fixation of graft within tunnels
7. Irrigation and closure of incisions

OPERATIVE NOTE
Preoperative Diagnosis: Anterior cruciate ligament-deficient knee

S. Saghieh et al. (eds.), *Operative Dictations in Orthopedic Surgery*,
DOI 10.1007/978-1-4614-7479-1_42,
© Springer Science+Business Media New York 2013

Procedure: ACL reconstruction using hamstring autograft
Postoperative Diagnosis: Same
Indications: ___ yo male/female who sustained a pivoting injury while playing basketball. She has had repeated episodes of instability and pain in the knee since that injury and wishes to return to cutting and pivoting sports. Clinically examination and an MRI confirmed an ACL rupture.
Description of Operation: The patient and surgical site were identified and marked. The patient underwent anesthesia per the anesthesia team. The patient was positioned supine on the operative table with all bony prominences padded. IV antibiotics were administered. An examination under anesthesia revealed a small effusion, positive Lachman's, pivot shift, and anterior drawer tests while posterior drawer and collateral ligament testing was normal. Soft roll and tourniquet cuff were placed about the right upper thigh, and the leg was then held by the thigh positioner. The right lower extremity was then sterilely prepped and draped in the standard surgical fashion. A time out was performed with the entire surgical, nursing, and anesthesia teams.

Anterolateral and anteromedial portals were developed on either side of the patellar tendon. The anterolateral portal was placed directly on the lateral aspect of the patella tendon. Care was taken to place the anteromedial portal using spinal needle guidance. The portal was placed medial and inferior enough so that anteromedial drilling of the femoral tunnel could later be performed. The outflow Veress needle was placed superomedially. A diagnostic arthroscopy of the knee joint was performed and the following findings were noted. The ACL was torn with a bare medial wall of the lateral condyle within the intercondylar notch. . The PCL was intact. The medial meniscus, medial femoral condyle, and medial tibial plateau were probed and normal. The lateral meniscus, lateral femoral condyle, and lateral tibial plateau were normal. The patella, trochlea, medial, and lateral gutters and the suprapatellar pouch were normal.

The notch was then visualized with the camera while the shaver was used to debride the stumps of the torn ACL and the center of the femoral and tibia footprints were marked using radiofrequency wand. The femoral ACL origin was debrided on the wall of the lateral femoral condyle so that the posterior aspect of the notch in the over-the-top position could be assessed. A minimal notchplasty was performed with a large shaver.

Attention was then turned to graft harvest. A vertical incision was made inferomedially directly over the pes anserinus insertion just medial to the tibial tubercle. The underlying soft tissues were sharply dissected to the level of the the sartorius fascia which was incised obliquely along the superior aspect of the pes tendons. The plane between the pes tendons and the superficial MCL was established. The fascial incision along the superior aspect of the pes tendons was then curved in a hockey stick fashion to detach the pes tendons from the tibia. The gracilis tendon was identified and was freed using Mayo scissors. A suture was placed in the free end of the gracilis and the semitendinosis tendons. The open ring graft harvester was placed, and the gracilis tendon harvested. Adhesions to the medial head of the gastrocnemius were freed from the semitendonosis which was also then harvested using the tendon stripper. The tendons were brought to the back table and remaining muscle was stripped away. The tendons were then quadrupled over a 20 mm Acufex Endobutton. The graft was 8 mm in diameter. The graft construct was placed on a tensioner under 15 lb of tension while the ACL tunnels were prepared.

Attention was then turned back to the arthroscopic portion of the case. The femoral footprint of the ACL was identified and a 5 mm over the top reference guide was placed such that the pin entered the center of the anatomic femoral footprint. The knee was hyperflexed to 110° and the Beath pin was advanced through the femur and out the skin of the distal lateral thigh. A 4.5 mm cannulated drill was used to drill through the femur with the lateral cortex being breached at 35 mm. An 8 mm acorn reamer was then drilled to a depth of 28 mm. A passing suture was placed through the femoral tunnel using the Beath pin. Bony debris from the drilling was suctioned away.

The tip pointed tibial guide was then placed in the center of the tibial footprint just lateral to the anterior tibial spine and in line with the posterior aspect of the anterior horn of the lateral meniscus. The guidepin was drilled through the tibia from the tibial incision to the tibial footprint. The knee was extended to confirm that there would not be impingement on the graft. A 8 mm tibial reamer was then used to create the tibial tunnel. A rasp was placed to chamfer the aperture of the tunnel into the joint. The passing suture loop that was placed in the femur was drawn down through the tibial tunnel.

The sutures of the Endobutton sutures were then looped through the passing suture loop and pulled up through the tibia and femur. The Endobutton sutures were then pulled to advance the ACL graft through the tibial tunnel and into femoral tunnel under endoscopic visualization. Once pulled all the way through, the Endobutton was deployed, and the graft was pulled taut distally, fixing the Endobutton on the femoral cortex. The graft was solid and was tensioned in flexion and extension repetitively. In full extension, the graft was arthroscopically assessed, and there was no impingement. The knee was then extended completely, and the graft tensioned. A 7–9 mm bioabsorbable soft tissue interference screw and sheath were advanced up the tibial tunnel with excellent fixation. The end of the stump was excised sharply. The graft was assessed again, moving the knee through a full range of motion, and it was noted to be solid. The knee was solid with grade 0 Lachman and grade 0 pivot.

The anteromedial incision was closed in layers with 0-Vicryl for the sartorial fascia, 2-0 Vicryl for subcutaneous tissue, 3-0 Monocryl running subcuticular and Steri-Strips for skin. Portals were closed with 3-0 Nylon. A sterile dressing and an Ace wrap were then placed. The patient was awakened and extubated and brought to the recovery room in stable condition with no immediate complications.

No intraoperative complications.

Staff was present and scrubbed for entire procedure.

Chapter 43
Anteromedial Tibia Tubercle Transfer

Said Saghieh, M.D.

COMMON INDICATIONS
Anterior knee pain associated with:
- Lateral patellar tilt
- Patellofemoral articular degeneration
- Recurrent subluxation
- Lateral patellar compression syndrome

POSSIBLE COMPLICATIONS
- Superficial or deep infection
- DVT
- Anterior compartment syndrome
- Fracture
- Nonunion
- Incisional neuroma
- Knee stiffness
- Failure to relieve pain
- Persistent or recurrent patellar instability

ESSENTIAL STEPS
1. Diagnostic arthroscopy
2. Anterolateral incision
3. Outline the osteotomy with drill holes
4. Complete osteotomy with a saw
5. Medial transfer
6. Fixation
7. Closure

S. Saghieh et al. (eds.), *Operative Dictations in Orthopedic Surgery*,
DOI 10.1007/978-1-4614-7479-1_43,
© Springer Science+Business Media New York 2013

OPERATIVE NOTE

Preoperative Diagnosis: Anterior knee pain secondary to patellofemoral maltracking

Procedure: Knee arthroscopy, Anteromedial tibial tubercle transfer

Postoperative Diagnosis: Same

Indications: This is a young woman who complains of anterior knee pain of year duration. Imaging studies are in favor of patellofemoral maltracking.

Description of Operation: Patient was identified in the preoperative holding area where marking of the extremity was performed. An IV was started. He was brought to the Operating Room and positioned supine on the operative table. General anesthetic was induced. IV antibiotics were given. A tourniquet was placed on the thigh. The left lower extremity was prepped and draped in the standard fashion.

A superomedial portal was made two finger breadths above the medial proximal pole of the patella. The patella articular cartilage was assessed as well as patella tracking. Findings confirmed the preoperative diagnosis. The scope was removed and the portal closed with nylon 4.0.

An anterolateral longitudinal incision was made lateral to the patellar tendon and was extended to a point 6 cm distal to the tibial tubercle at the anterior midline.

The patellar tendon was identified and a lateral retinacular release was performed.

The patella was partially everted and its articular surface inspected.

The periosteum was incised longitudinally from the medial side of the crest for 10 cm. Similarly, the lateral side of the patella was exposed by dissecting off the anterior compartment musculature.

A 9/64-in. drill bit was used to create multiple parallel holes starting medially at an oblique angle and exiting the lateral cortex more posterior under direct vision. The osteotomy was outlined in a fashion where the pedicle of bone deep to the tibial tubercle was fairly thick and tapered anteriorly to reach 2 mm distally. It had a length of 8 cm.

An oscillating saw was used to complete the osteotomy. The bone pedicle was advanced anteromedially along the osteotomy plane.

Two parallel anteroposterior cortical 4.5 mm lag screws were used to fix the pedicle.

The wound was heavily irrigated and closed in anatomical layers; the subcutaneous tissue with vicryl 2.0 and the skin with staplers.

A sterile dressing was applied.

Surgical staff was present.

Chapter 44
Lateral Retinacular Release

Said Saghieh, M.D.

COMMON INDICATIONS
- Recurrent subluxation
- Chondromalacia of the patella
- Tight lateral structures
- Lateral tilt with minimal lateral subluxation on roentgenogram in combination with realignment procedure
- Lateral patellar compression syndrome

POSSIBLE COMPLICATIONS
- Failure to relieve pain
- Patellar instability/dislocation

ESSENTIAL STEPS
1. Diagnostic arthroscopy
2. Examine Patella tracking
3. Divide retinaculum
4. Confirm release

OPERATIVE NOTE
Preoperative Diagnosis: Patella subluxation, R/L
Procedure: Lateral Retinacular Release
Postoperative Diagnosis: Same
Indications: This is a young M/F who has been complaining of anterior knee pain associated with painful episodes of patella subluxation
Description of Operation: Patient was identified and the affected extremity was marked in the preoperative holding area. An IV was

S. Saghieh et al. (eds.), *Operative Dictations in Orthopedic Surgery*,
DOI 10.1007/978-1-4614-7479-1_44,
© Springer Science+Business Media New York 2013

started. He was brought to the Operating Room and positioned supine on the operative table. General anesthetic was induced. IV antibiotics were given. A tourniquet was placed on the right/left leg that was prepped and draped in the standard fashion. A standard lateral infrapatellar portal was made. The arthroscope was introduced and a diagnostic arthroscopy performed (Findings). The medial infrapatellar portal was made under direct visualization. A superolateral portal was then created through which a 70° arthroscope was inserted.

The patellar tracking was observed and obvious lateral tracking of the patella was noted. The patella did not centralize until approximately __ degrees of knee flexion. Approximately ___ of the patella remained lateral to the lateral aspect of the trochlea at the terminal 45° extension. The trochlear groove appeared shallow throughout all of its depth and extension. The intracondylar notch was inspected and the cruciate ligaments were found to be intact without evidence of injury. The inferior edge of the vastus lateralis tendon was palpated. Junction marked at its insertion into the patella with an 18-gauge spinal needle at the superior pole of the patella. A coblator knife was inserted into the anterolateral portal, and under arthroscopic guidance it divided the synovium and lateral retinaculum from the superolateral corner of the patella to the inferior extent of the lateral border of the patellar tendon. The release was extended proximally along the lateral border of the vastus lateralis tendon. Following this the patella was tilted about 90° perpendicular to the notch to confirm release. 3.0 nylon was then used to close the portal incisions.

A bandage was applied. The tourniquet was deflated. The patient was extubated and transferred to the recovery room.

A staff was present and scrubbed for the entire procedure.

Chapter 45

Chronic/Exertional Compartment Syndrome Release

Michael J. Huang, M.D.

COMMON INDICATIONS

- Pain that is gradual in onset during exercise, ultimately restricting performance that fails conservative therapy.
- Compartment pressures taken before, during, after exercise (pressures >15 mmHg fifteen minutes after exercise, or absolute values above 15 mmHg while resting or above 30 mmHg after exercise).

POSSIBLE COMPLICATIONS

- Neurologic damage
- Vascular damage
- Incomplete release
- Wound complications (i.e., infection, dehiscence)

ESSENTIAL STEPS

1. Two skin incisions: one proximal and one distal in line with anterolateral intermuscular septum
2. Identify fascia
3. Look for superficial peroneal nerve
4. Incise fascia between incisions
5. Irrigate and obtain hemostasis
6. Close

OPERATIVE NOTE

Preoperative Diagnosis: Rt/Lt exertional compartment syndrome

Procedure: Rt/Lt exertional compartment syndrome release

S. Saghieh et al. (eds.), *Operative Dictations in Orthopedic Surgery*,
DOI 10.1007/978-1-4614-7479-1_45,
© Springer Science+Business Media New York 2013

Postoperative Diagnosis: Same

Indications: __ -year-old man/woman who complains of anterior shin pain upon exertion. The pain continually progresses as he/she continues with activity and is relieved with stopping these activities. Traditional methods of rest and nonsteroidals were not effective. Compartments were measured in the clinic and at rest were in the 10 s to 20 s in the anterior and lateral as well as posterior compartments. Upon exertion, however, the compartments were measured again in the 50 s and 60 s in the anterior compartments. All other compartments were within normal levels. Therefore, patient elected to undergo anterior compartment fasciotomy. Risks and benefits of this procedure were discussed with the patient and informed consent was obtained.

Description of Operation:

Patient was taken to the operating room and was placed in the supine position. General anesthesia was induced by the Anesthesia staff. Thigh tourniquet was placed. Rt/Lt lower extremity was then prepped and draped in the normal sterile fashion.

Starting at the midpoint between the anterior tibial crest and the fibula, two 5–6 cm incisions were made, one proximal and one distal in line with the anterolateral intramuscular septum. The septum was then identified beginning with the distal portion over the middle to distal one-third. An incision was made in the anterior fascia. The superficial peroneal nerve was visualized at this point. It was noted to be intact and protected throughout the procedure. The fascial incision was then carried distally to the level of the peroneal tendons. It was then carried proximally to the extent of the incision. Through the more proximal incision the fascia was again identified and incision was made in the fascia and carried down to the previous incision in the distal portion of the wound. The fascia was directly visualized throughout its course. The fascia was then split proximally up to the level of the tibiofibular joint. The wound was then irrigated and closed using 2-0 Vicryl sutures in the subcutaneous layer and running Nylon suture in the skin.

Tourniquet was/or was not inflated during the procedure. There were no complications and patient was taken to the recovery room in stable condition.

Dr. ____ was present and scrubbed for the entire case.

Chapter 46

Tibia Intramedullary Nail

John-Erik Bell, M.D., M.S.

COMMON INDICATIONS
- Tibial shaft diaphyseal fractures

POSSIBLE COMPLICATIONS
- Anterior knee pain (up to 50 %)
- Neurovascular injury
- Compartment syndrome
- Intra-articular fracture propogation
- Thermal necrosis with reaming
- Nonunion
- Malunion
- Infection

ESSENTIAL STEPS
1. Positioning—supine on either the fracture table (leg at 90, traction through calcaneus pin or skin, pad under popliteal fossa) or supine on radiolucent table (manual traction, leg flexed to 90 over radiolucent triangle).
2. Check fluoro visualization of entire tibia and adequacy of reduction before prepping (be sure to note rotational alignment).
3. Starting point—preferably extraarticular just beneath joint line, medial to patellar tendon (unless a very proximal fracture—then go lateral), line up between tibial spines or in line with lateral spine.

S. Saghieh et al. (eds.), *Operative Dictations in Orthopedic Surgery*,
DOI 10.1007/978-1-4614-7479-1_46,
© Springer Science+Business Media New York 2013

4. Open medullary canal with cannulated drill or awl.
5. Guide wire down canal, checking AP and lateral alignment, take care to make sure wire is centered well in distal fragment.
6. Measure nail length and diameter.
7. Overream by 2.0 mm.
8. Place nail over guide wire.
9. Proximally lock the nail with targeting device.
10. Distally cross lock using freehand perfect circles technique.

OPERATIVE NOTE
Preoperative Diagnosis: Tibial diaphyseal fracture
Procedure: Tibial intramedullary nail
Postoperative Diagnosis: Same
Description of Operation: The patient was identified and the site of surgery confirmed. Anesthesia was induced. Prophylactic IV antibiotics were administered. The patient was placed supine on a radiolucent operating table, a padded thigh tourniquet was placed, the leg was shaved, and all bony prominences were padded. Fluoroscopy was brought in to confirm visualization of the entire tibia in the AP and lateral planes and a closed reduction was performed. Alignment was confirmed with fluoroscopy and the patient was prepped and draped.

A longitudinal incision measuring 3 cm was made over the patellar tendon. Dissection was carried through the subcutaneous tissues to the fascia. The fascia was incised just medial to the patellar tendon and the periosteum of the proximal tibia exposed. The threaded guide wire was positioned on the AP between the tibial spines in line with the long axis of the tibia, and on the lateral, directed parallel with the anterior cortex. The canal was then opened with the cannulated drill over the guide wire. The fracture was then closed reduced. The ball-tipped reaming guide wire was then inserted down the canal through the fracture site and into the distal fragment, taking care to center the wire in the distal fragment. The length of the nail was then measured. The canal was reamed sequentially, stopping after overreaming the measured nail diameter by 2.0 mm. Over the guide wire, the cannulated tibial nail was inserted, monitoring passage through the fracture site to ensure alignment. The guide wire was then removed.

Then, using the proximal targeting device, the proximal cross-locking screws were inserted and placement confirmed fluoroscopically. Then using the freehand perfect circles technique, the distal cross-locking screws were inserted and confirmed fluoroscopically. All wounds were irrigated thoroughly, the deep fascia approximated with 0-vicryl, the subcutaneous tissues with 2-0 vicryl, and the skin with staples. Dressings were applied. No complications were encountered and the patient was awakened and taken to recovery in stable condition. Postoperative plan includes weight-bearing as tolerated and knee range of motion.

Chapter 47

Meniscus Repair

Brian R. Wolf, M.D., M.S.

COMMON INDICATIONS

- Vertical longitudinal tears in the peripheral red-red or red-white zones of the meniscus.

POSSIBLE COMPLICATIONS

- Failure of meniscal healing
- Saphenous nerve or vein injury
- Peroneal nerve injury
- Infection
- Thrombophlebitis

ESSENTIAL STEPS

1. Supine positioning.
2. Diagnostic knee arthroscopy and identification of meniscal tear.
3. Gentle debridement and rasping of the edges of the meniscal tear and surrounding capsule to stimulate bleeding.
4. Repair of meniscal tear using chosen technique.
5. Probe meniscus to test repair.
6. Wound irrigation and closure.

S. Saghieh et al. (eds.), *Operative Dictations in Orthopedic Surgery*,
DOI 10.1007/978-1-4614-7479-1_47,
© Springer Science+Business Media New York 2013

OPERATIVE NOTE

Preoperative Diagnosis: Peripheral meniscal tear in vertical longitudinal orientation

Procedure: Knee arthroscopy, medial meniscus repair

Postoperative Diagnosis: Same

Indications: __ yo male or female with knee joint line tenderness and mechanical symptoms with a suspected meniscus tear.

Description of Operation: The patient was taken to the operating room and placed in the supine position. Anesthesia was induced. Examination under anesthesia demonstrated full range of motion, no effusion, and stable collateral and cruciate ligaments. A tourniquet was placed over the left thigh. The left leg was then placed into the leg holder. The left lower extremity was then prepped and draped in the normal sterile fashion. A multidisciplinary time-out was performed confirming the correct patient, procedure, and extremity.

An anterolateral parapatellar portal was established and the camera inserted. A superomedial outflow portal with a Veress needle was made. Under needle localization an anteromedial portal was established.

A diagnostic arthroscopy was performed with the following findings. The patellofemoral joint was noted to be normal without any areas of chondromalacia of the trochlea or patella. The suprapatellar pouch, medial gutter, and lateral gutter were normal. The lateral compartment was next visualized. The lateral meniscus was noted to be normal. There was no chondromalacia noted of the lateral femoral condyle or lateral tibial plateau. The ACL and PCL were also noted to be normal.

The camera was then placed into the medial compartment. Upon entering the medial compartment, a peripheral meniscal tear was visualized. It was at the red-red junction along the area of the meniscocapsular junction posteriorly and measured 20 mm in medial to lateral length. The meniscus could be drawn into the joint. A shaver and rasp were then placed into the tear area to debride the edge of the meniscus and to stimulate bleeding from the surrounding synovium in the area. The camera was then placed along the femoral notch and into the posterior aspect of the medial compartment. The medial meniscus was clearly visualized with the scope extended into this area. This area was also debrided to stimulate bleeding. A FasT-Fix anchor system was then used to secure the meniscus to the peripheral capsule using vertical sutures across the tear. Three FasT-fix sutures were used. Once this was completed, a probe was used to test the meniscus, and it was noted to be stable and well opposed. There were no complications with the procedure. The portals were closed with Nylon sutures and sterile dressings were applied.

Staff was present for entire procedure.

Chapter 48
Standard Below Knee Amputation

Anthony V. Mollano, M.D.

COMMON INDICATIONS
- Combination of peripheral vascular disease, osteomyelitis, diabetes, peripheral neuropathy
- Charcot osteoarthropathy
- Traumatized lower extremity with severe neurovascular injury
- Malignancy
- Failure of a more distal amputation
- Congenital deformity

POSSIBLE COMPLICATIONS
- Early (Mortality from sepsis > heart disease
- Morbidity from pneumonia > heart disease
- Depression
- Wound infection
- Hematoma
- Wound dehiscence
- Delayed wound healing
- Gangrene of stump
- Necrosis of skin margins
- Pressure necrosis
- Edema
- Pain
- Contracture
- Late (Phantom pain; Neuroma; Bursitis; RSD; Late stump problems from skin disorders, redundant soft tissue, and bone problems)

S. Saghieh et al. (eds.), *Operative Dictations in Orthopedic Surgery*,
DOI 10.1007/978-1-4614-7479-1_48,
© Springer Science+Business Media New York 2013

ESSENTIAL STEPS

1. Administer anesthesia.
2. Place ankle in a bag after proper supine positioning on the table.
3. Sterilely prep and drape.
4. Exsanguinate leg by gravity and pneumotourniquet.
5. In long posterior flap technique, make an anterior incision on the leg slightly distal to the intended tibial bone cut (12.5–17.5 cm below the medial knee joint line) and end at about two-thirds of the circumference of the leg; then extend the lateral and medial limbs of the incision about 2.5 cm longer than the diameter of the leg at the anterior incision; and finish the cuts by turning them posterior to finish the posterior flap (allowing for a posterior flap length that is at least two-thirds of the AP diameter of the calf at the level of the intended tibial bone cut).
6. Carry the anterior incision through all tissues to bone, and identify anterior tibial nerve and superficial peroneal nerve so that the vessel could be properly clamped/ligated, and the nerve could be transected under traction.
7. Incise and elevate the periosteum, and then transect the tibia with power saw, or Gigli saw, beveling its anterior aspect.
8. Transect fibula 1 cm proximal to the level of tibial cut.
9. Draw amputation knife distally and posteriorly to create thick beveled myocutaneous flap, followed by transection of deep posterior muscles leaving gastrocnemius and soleus as the myofascial flap.
10. Deliver amputated leg off the table.
11. Identify neurovascular structures, clamp/ligate vessels, and transect nerves under traction (deep peroneal, tibial, superficial peroneal, saphenous, lateral sural cutaneous).
12. Bevel and smooth bone edges; trim posterior flap mass.
13. Reverse tourniquet and assure hemostasis.
14. Irrigate with pulsatile lavage; close fascia well with good apposition of fascia under tension, allowing closure of skin without tension using interrupted nonabsorbable material; apply a sterile, dry dressing.

OPERATIVE NOTE

Preoperative Diagnosis: Foot and ankle open crush injury
Procedure: Below knee amputation
Postoperative Diagnosis: Same

Indications: This is an X-year-old patient with an open foot and ankle crush injury with diffuse ischemia and anesthesia. Amputation is indicated to facilitate ambulation and rehabilitation. Patient understood risks and benefits of below knee amputation, and elected to proceed.

Description of Operation: After anesthesia was delivered, the foot was placed in Lahey bag, and the leg was sterilely prepped and draped. It was exsanguinated by gravity and a pneumotourniquet was inflated at the level of the thigh for thirty minutes using 350 mmHg. A standard incision was made on the anterior aspect of the leg 15 cm below medial joint line, extended laterally and medially, and then posteriorly to finish the posterior flap. The subcutaneous tissue was cut to the level of the fascia, and then incised. The anterior vessel bleeders were identified, and tied off with 2-0 silk, and the residual nerves were transected high into the flaps. The tibia was identified and transected about 5 mm proximal to the skin line, and the anterior aspect of the tibia was beveled. The anterior musculature was incised, and the fibula was identified and transected about 1 cm proximal to the level of tibial cut. The amputation knife was utilized to transect the remaining soft tissue and finish the posterior flap. The distal leg was delivered off the table. Working from anterior to posterior, major vessel bleeders were identified, and tied off with 2-0 silk, and the residual nerves were transected high into the flaps. The tourniquet was reversed and good hemostasis was achieved. The stump was irrigated with 1.5 L of pulsatile lavage, and closed in a layered fashion using 0 Vicryl, 2-0 Vicryl, 2-0 Proline, and 3-0 Nylon. A clean, sterile, dry dressing was applied, and the patient was taken to the recovery room in good condition. Sponge and instrument counts were correct at the end of the case, times two. Dr. Staff Attending Surgeon was present, scrubbed, and participated actively in all aspects of the procedure.

Chapter 49

Tibia Shaft Angular Deformity Correction by TSF

Said Saghieh, M.D.

COMMON INDICATIONS
- Midshaft leg deformity (usually posttraumatic)

POSSIBLE COMPLICATIONS
- Deep or superficial infection
- Compartment syndrome
- Neurovascular injury or entrapment by wire placement
- Nonunion
- Under- or over correction

ESSENTIAL STEPS
1. Preoperative planning to determine the CORA and the placement of the frame.
2. Preoperative construct of the frame with the available software.
3. Prepping and draping of the leg.
4. Application of the frame with the reference ring orthogonal to the bone in both planes.
5. Percutaneous osteotomy at the desired preplanned point (usually the CORA).
6. Closure.

OPERATIVE NOTE
Preoperative Diagnosis: Midshaft leg deformity
Procedure: Percutaneous tibia osteotomy and application of TSF (Taylor Spatial Frame)

S. Saghieh et al. (eds.), *Operative Dictations in Orthopedic Surgery*,
DOI 10.1007/978-1-4614-7479-1_49,

Postoperative Diagnosis: Same

Indication: ---year-old male/female patient with midshaft tibia deformity of -- degrees.

Description of Operation: The patient was identified in the preoperative holding area and the extremity was marked.

The patient was brought to the operating room and positioned supine on the operating table. General (or regional) anesthesia was induced by the anesthesiologist. All pressure points were well padded. A padded sand bag was applied under the right/left buttock. Prophylactic IV antibiotics (name and dose) were administered. The extremity was prepped and draped in a sterile fashion.

The preoperative constructed TSF was applied over the leg. We made sure about the ring sizes and the circumferential soft-tissue clearance.

The first half pin was applied in the proximal fragment 3 finger breadths proximal to the apex of deformity just medial to the shin and in an anteroposterior direction. Its position was confirmed by fluoroscopy to be perpendicular to the bone.

The pin was connected to the upper surface of the proximal ring making sure that the master tab was anterior and centered over the bone. A two-hole cube was attached to the proximal ring over the anteromedial side of the bone through which a second half pin was applied perpendicular to the bone under fluoroscopy control. The placement of these two half pins determined the orthogonal placement of the proximal ring over the tibia. A third half pin was added on the anteromedial side of the bone inferior to the proximal ring. Its position was checked not to interfere with the struts.

The distal ring position was checked under fluoroscopy and was considered to be satisfactory. (It should be orthogonal or slightly off. If the position is not satisfied, the surgeon has to change the configuration using the software or disconnect the struts, apply the distal ring in an orthogonal fashion over the bone, reconnect the struts, and then run the total residual program.)

The ring was fixed to the bone by three half pins; one proximal on the anteromedial side of the bone; and two distal half pins (one is anterior and one is anteromedial).

A 2.5 cm longitudinal skin incision was performed over the apex of the deformity (or over the preplanned osteotomy side if different) on the anteromedial side of the tibia. It was deepened to the periosteum. An elevator was used to peel off the periosteum circumferentially. A 2.5 mm drill bit centered in a sleeve was used to perform multiple holes at the site of the preplanned osteotomy that was completed with the use of 2 cm osteotome. All six struts were disconnected and the osteotomy was checked under fluoroscopy to be complete. The wound was closed anatomically in two layers: the subcutaneous layer with vicryl 2.0 and the skin with staples. The struts were again connected. The fluoroscopy confirmed good apposition of the two fragments with no gap.

A sterile dressing was applied and the fixator was wrapped with elastic bandage. The patient was awakened from anesthesia and was transported to the recovery room in satisfactory condition. There were no immediate complications associated with the procedure (or list complication and describe treatment or action taken, if any). Staff was present and scrubbed for entire procedure.

Chapter 50

Mini-Invasive Primary Total Knee Arthroplasty

Said Saghieh, M.D.

COMMON INDICATIONS

- Primary or secondary osteoarthritis of the knee.
- Rheumatoid arthritis.
- Arthropathy secondary to hemophilia.
- Malalignment producing asymmetric wearing of the knee.
- All leading to significant impairment of ambulation and failing to respond to more conservative treatment.

POSSIBLE COMPLICATIONS

- Infection
- Thromboembolic phenomenon
- Neurocirculatory compromise
- Fracture dislocation
- Stiffness
- Patellar problems
- Late loosening

ESSENTIAL STEPS

1. Templating of radiographs
2. Placement and inflation of tourniquet
3. Incision of skin and soft tissues
4. Medial arthrotomy
5. Release of the medial meniscus
6. Distal femoral cuts
7. Tibial cuts
8. Placement of trial components
9. Placement of permanent components

S. Saghieh et al. (eds.), *Operative Dictations in Orthopedic Surgery*,
DOI 10.1007/978-1-4614-7479-1_50,
© Springer Science+Business Media New York 2013

10. Closure of the arthrotomy
11. Closure of skin and soft tissue
12. Placement in bulky dressing or knee immobilizer

OPERATIVE NOTE

Preoperative Diagnosis: Knee osteoarthritis
Procedure: Cemented total knee replacement
Postoperative Diagnosis: Knee osteoarthritis
Indication: The patient is a ___-year-old male/female with severe knee pain and difficulty with ambulation secondary to osteoarthritis.
Description of Operation:
Implants Used:
Femoral:
Tibial Tray:
Polyethylene:
The patient was brought into the operating room and placed in a supine position. General endotracheal anesthesia was performed by the anesthesia team. The patient was given prophylactic antibiotics, a Foley was inserted, and the tourniquet was applied. All extremities were well padded. The leg was prepped and draped for surgery. The tourniquet was inflated to 350 mmHg. A slightly oblique median parapatellar 10 cm skin incision was carried out starting at the superior pole of the patella to end at the center of the tibial tubercle. The incision was carried through the subcutaneous tissue. A median parapatellar arthrotomy was performed. It was carried proximally to the superior pole of the patella where the vastus medialis was identified and split for 2–3 cm. Distally, the tibial tendon was dissected off the proximal tibia to its insertion at the tibia tubercle that was left intact.

The knee was extended to 20°. The Hoffa's fad pad was resected and the patella was subluxed laterally. The anterior horn of the medial meniscus was detached and varus release was performed as necessary. The ACL was cut and debrided. The anterior horn of the lateral meniscus was also removed.

The knee was flexed to 90°. An 8 mm drill was used to open the femoral canal. The distal femoral cutting jig was then placed in 5–6° of valgus as measured on the preoperative scanogram. 9 mm of the medial condyle and 7 mm of the lateral condyle were removed (the values may be different in valgus femur and may increase in the presence of flexion contracture where additional 2 mm need to be resected from both sides).

The anterior tibia was exposed. The extra-medullary proximal tibial cutting jig was placed. The ankle strap was tightened.

The alignment guide was checked to be 5–10 mm medial to the center of the intermalleoli distance, parallel to the tibia shin, and overlying the medial third of the tibia tubercle. The alignment guide was manipulated to be parallel to the tibia axis in the sagital plane as well. Its height was adjusted to get a minimal cut from the medial plateau (in varus knee) or 10 mm cut from the lateral plateau. The cutting jig was fixed to the bone. The guide was removed and proximal tibia resection was performed.

Extension gap was then measured. It accommodated 10 mm spacer and was symmetrical.

The alignment was also checked and was satisfactory.

The remnants of the menisci and the cruciate ligaments were excised.

The femoral sizing guide was then applied. The locking anterior boom was set on the highest point of the lateral cortex. The appropriate size was selected. The epicondylar axis was then identified and the correct rotational plate applied.

Femur anterior and posterior cuts and chamfers were performed as well as the trochlear recess cuts.

Flexion gap was measured. It was equal to the extension gap (10 mm) and symmetrical.

Finally, the femoral intercondylar box was prepared.

The tibia surface was measured and the appropriate tray was selected (– – –).

The femoral component and tibial component were placed. The patient came to full extension and flexed to 130°. Rotation for the tibia was set at this time. The components were removed. The tibial drill followed by the punch was set into the tibia.

The patella was measured to be ___ mm. It was osteotomized to ___ mm. Three drill holes were placed in the patella. The patellar trial component was placed. The thickness between patella and component was ___ mm.

A thorough irrigation was performed while cement was mixed and applied to the selected components prepared on the field.

The knee was brought into flexion. The femoral component was placed followed directly by the tibial component. Excessive cement was removed. A – – –mm trial spacer was inserted and the knee was brought out into extension. Cement was pressurized into the patella. The patellar component was applied. The patellar clamp was applied. Residual cement was removed.

After the cement settled, the range of motion was again examined (0–130°). The patella tracked well. The selected polyethylene was inserted. The tourniquet was deflated. Hemostasis was achieved with electrocautery. A hemovac drain was placed deep coming through the anterolateral skin. The arthrotomy and the vastus medialis were closed with #1 Vicryl. 2-0 Vicryl interrupted sutures were used for subcutaneous closure. Skin was closed with staplers. The patient was awakened, placed on the hospital bed, and taken to the recovery room in satisfactory condition.

Postoperative activity restrictions: Early range of motion using a continuous passive motion machine. Extension should be achieved early and flexion should be at 90° by the time of discharge from the hospital. Patient may be partial weight bearing on the first postoperative day and use a knee immobilizer until sufficient quadriceps strength has returned.

There were no intraoperative complications.

Total tourniquet time was _____.

Faculty was present for the entire procedure.

Chapter 51
Open Reduction and Internal Fixation of Tibial Plateau Fractures

Hamdi G. Sukkarieh, M.D.

COMMON INDICATIONS
Absolute Indications
- Open plateau fractures
- Fractures with an associated compartment syndrome
- Fractures with a vascular injury

Relative Indications
- Most displaced bicondylar fractures
- Displaced medial condyle fractures
- Coronal-plane posterior condylar fracture-dislocations
- Lateral plateau fractures that result in axial joint instability

POSSIBLE COMPLICATIONS
- Early wound breakdown
- Infection
- Septic arthritis
- Painful hardware
- Loss of fixation
- Nonunion
- Malunion
- Knee stiffness
- Posttraumatic arthritis
- Heterotopic ossification
- Thromboembolic complications

S. Saghieh et al. (eds.), *Operative Dictations in Orthopedic Surgery*,
DOI 10.1007/978-1-4614-7479-1_51,
© Springer Science+Business Media New York 2013

ESSENTIAL STEPS

1. General or spinal anesthesia.
2. Positioning: supine on a radiolucent operating table.
3. Large bolster or a bean bag patient positioner under the ipsilateral hip.
4. C-arm image intensifier is positioned on the contralateral side.
5. Trial images should be obtained prior to prepping and draping to ensure that accurate AP, lateral, and oblique fluoroscopic images are easily attainable without interference.
6. If an iliac crest bone graft is planned, then the ipsilateral crest is also included in the initial prep and a sterile tourniquet is utilized.
7. Contemporary implants include 2.7- and 3.5-mm low profile sizes, which are precontoured to match the proximal tibial condylar anatomy.
8. The large 4.5- and 6.5-mm implants are used less frequently today.
9. Skin incisions for tibial plateau fractures should be longitudinal and as close to the midline as possible.
10. The plane of dissection over the anterior patella should be below the fascia, which supplies blood to the prepatellar skin.
11. Apply a tourniquet except in patients with severe soft-tissue injury.

OPERATIVE NOTE

Preoperative Diagnosis: Tibial plateau fracture, schatzker III
Procedure: Open reduction and internal fixation of tibial plateau fracture, scatzker III
Postoperative Diagnosis: Same
Indications: This is a ——-year-old M/F who sustained a tibial plateau fracture, scatzker III
Description of Operation: The patient was identified and the affected site confirmed. Under GA or spinal anesthesia with the patient in the supine position on a radiolucent table, with a bolster under the ipsilateral hip and a proximal thigh tourniquet, the affected lower extremity was shaved, prepped, and draped in the usual sterile fashion. Prophylactic intravenous antibiotics were given. The tourniquet was inflated. A small lateral incision was made over the metaphyseal region of the lateral condyle, and exposure was limited to develop a small, subcondylar, metaphyseal,

cortical window. A periosteal elevator was introduced well beneath the depressed articular fragments and the articular fragments and compressed cancellous bone were elevated in one large mass. The resulting void was filled with cancellous bone graft, which was then packed snugly using an inlay impactor. The fracture was held with a large pointed forceps placed percutaneously on the medial and lateral condyles to compress the fracture line. The fragments were temporarily fixed with multiple small Kirschner wires. Fixation was accomplished with two or three 6.5- or 7.0-mm screws placed through small stab incisions, or occasionally through use of multiple 3.5-mm cortical screws, cannulated or non-cannulated. Adequacy of reduction was confirmed by fluoroscopy. The wound was heavily irrigated. The deep fascia was approximated with 0-vicryl, the subcutaneous tissues with 2-0 vicryl, and the skin with staples. Dressings were applied. No complications were encountered and the patient was awakened and taken to recovery in stable condition.

Postoperative Management: Postoperatively, the limb is placed into a bulky dressing. A cephalosporin is administered for 24–48 h. A suction drain is maintained for at least 24 h or until drainage is less than 30 mL per 8 h interval. If the soft-tissue envelope was not significantly damaged at the time of injury and wound closure was achieved without tension, a continuous passive motion (CPM) machine is recommended. If significant swelling or tension on the suture line is present, the CPM is delayed until the swelling has subsided. The bulky dressing is removed at 48 h and a hinged knee brace that allows gradual increase in range of motion is applied. If a meniscal tear was present and repaired, the range of motion is usually limited for the first 3 weeks with flexion stops at 60 degrees. This protects the peripheral meniscal rim and allows early healing prior to initiation of full, unrestricted range of motion. Physical therapy is initiated early to begin quadriceps strengthening as well as non-weight-bearing gait training with crutches or a walker. Patients are seen at 2 weeks for suture removal and at monthly intervals thereafter. Once the wound is healed, active and active-assisted range of motion is initiated. The goal is to achieve at least 90° of knee flexion by the fourth week after surgery. Weight bearing of up to 50 % of body weight is initiated at 8–12 weeks if radiographic evidence show subchondral healing, metaphyseal consolidation, and incorporation of the subchondral void; this evidence is especially important when bone graft or bone graft substitutes have been utilized to fill the subchondral defect.

Part V
Foot and Ankle

Chapter 52

Hallux Valgus–Proximal Ludloff Osteotomy

Said Saghieh, M.D.

COMMON INDICATIONS

- Symptomatic hallux valgus with an intermetatarsal angle of greater than 14° and a hallux valgus angle greater than 35°.
- Patient without significant degenerative arthritis in the first metatarsophalangeal joint.

POSSIBLE COMPLICATIONS

- The distal fragment tends to displace dorsally or migrate medially to its original position unless securely fixed internally.
- The immediate convalescence usually is characterized by more pain, swelling, and immobility than that which follows a distally placed osteotomy.
- Hallux varus.

ESSENTIAL STEPS

1. Distal release of adductor hallucis, the deep transverse intermetatarsal ligament, and the lateral capsule of the first metatarsophalangeal joint.
2. Medial incision, careful to avoid neurovascular structures.
3. Drill, tap, and countersink distal hole prior to osteotomy.
4. Oblique osteotomy of proximal metatarsal.

S. Saghieh et al. (eds.), *Operative Dictations in Orthopedic Surgery*,
DOI 10.1007/978-1-4614-7479-1_52,
© Springer Science+Business Media New York 2013

5. Reduction of distal fragment.
6. First screw compression fixation.
7. Second lag screw fixation.

OPERATIVE NOTE
Preoperative Diagnosis: Hallux valgus
Procedure: Ludloff proximal metatarsal osteotomy
Postoperative Diagnosis: Same
Indication: This is a ____-year-old female who is complaining of R/L painful bunion associated with difficulty in shoe wear.
Description of Operation: The patient was identified and the site of the surgery was marked in the holding area. He/she was brought to the operating room and placed supine on the operating table. Regional anesthesia was induced and 1 g of Ancef was administered intravenously. A thigh tourniquet was applied and inflated to 250 mmHg after the foot was prepped and draped in the usual sterile fashion.

A longitudinal 2 cm incision was performed in the first web space. The adductor tendon was identified and released from its insertion on the lateral aspect of the proximal phalanx. Next, the metatarsal–sesamoid and intermetatarsal ligaments were released and the lateral capsule fenestrated at the joint line with a varus force applied to the hallux.

Next, attention was directed to the medial side of the foot. A midline longitudinal incision was made on the medial side of the foot extending from the base of the first metatarsal to the proximal phalanx distally. Local neurovascular structures were identified and retracted. An L-shaped capsulotomy with distal plantar apex was performed.

The medial eminence was exposed and resected with the cut performed 1 mm medial to the sagittal sulcus parallel to the metatarsal axis.

Then, Ludloff osteotomy was planned carefully to start dorsally 3 mm from the metarsal-cuneiform joint and extends distally at an angle of approximately 30° to the shaft of the metatarsal so that it exits the plantar cortex, just proximal to the sesamoids.

Prior to doing the osteotomy, I carefully drilled, tapped, and placed in a 3.5 partially threaded headless screw. The screw was perpendicular to the planned osteotomy. The screw was pulled out from the distal fragment before the osteotomy was performed with a sagittal saw. Then the screw was reinserted but not tightened at this stage.

After, I reduced the first metatarsal head under fluoroscopic guidance and fixed the first and second metatarsals with a single pin, the correction was checked fluoroscopically and then the screw was fully tightened to compress the osteotomy. A second similar screw was placed from plantar to dorsal parallel and distal to the first screw.

The residual overhanging medial ridge on the proximal segment was resected with the saw. The medial capsule was then imbricated while the hallux was held in a neutral or slightly abducted position.

After thourough irrigation, the wound was closed in a layered fashion, using 2-0 Vicryl for the subcutaneous tissue and 4-0 Nylon for the skin. A clean, sterile, dry dressing was applied and the patient was taken to the Recovery Room in good condition.

Dr___was present and scrubbed during the procedure.

Chapter 53
Distal Chevron Osteotomy with Capsulorrhaphy

Rola H. Rashid, M.D.

COMMON INDICATIONS
- Painful hallux valgus deformity recalcitrant to nonoperative measures and wishes to undergo operative fixation.

POSSIBLE COMPLICATIONS
- Anesthesia
- Paresthesias
- Infection
- Recurrent deformity

ESSENTIAL STEPS
1. Incision laterally to release tight structures.
2. Medial incision for exostectomy
3. Chevron osteotomy followed by stabilization of osteotomy
4. Wound closure

OPERATIVE NOTE
Preoperative Diagnosis: Hallux valgus
Procedure: Distal chevron osteotomy with capulorrhaphy
Postoperative Diagnosis: Same
Description of Operation: Patient was identified in the preoperative holding area, brought to the operative, and placed on the operative table in the supine position. The appropriate lower extremity was identified and confirmed. After induction of anesthesia, the extremity was prepped and draped in the usual sterile fashion.

S. Saghieh et al. (eds.), *Operative Dictations in Orthopedic Surgery*, DOI 10.1007/978-1-4614-7479-1_53,

A tourniquet was placed on the shin over several layers of cast padding. An esmarch was used to exsanguinate the extremity. The tourniquet was then inflated to 250 mmHg.

We first directed attention to the first web space where a longitudinal 2 cm incision was performed. The adductor tendon was identified and released from its insertion on the lateral aspect of the proximal phalanx. Next, the metatarsal–sesamoid and inter-metatarsal ligaments were released and the lateral capsule fenestrated at the joint line with a varus force applied to the hallux.

Then a 5 cm incision was made medially, centered over the MTP joint. A sharp dissection was carried through the subcutaneous layers with care taken to protect the neural structures. The capsule was identified and then incised longitudinally the length of the incision. The plantar and dorsal flaps were then created with sharp dissection. The MTP was identified. Homan retractors were placed. Medial exostectomy was performed. Next attention was turned to planning the chevron osteotomy. The plantar cut was made virtually parallel to the floor. Then at about a 70–80° angle the dorsal limb was made. A towel clip was used to grab the proximal fragment and the distal fragment was manipulated. Excellent clinical alignment was achieved and the osteotomy was held using standard technique for a bioabsorbable pin. This was drilled, first secured with a K-wire, stabilized, trialed, and then put in place.

The wound was then copiously irrigated. Repair and medial tightening of the capsule was performed with 2-0 Vicryl. Skin was closed using Monocryl and Steri-Strips. Bunion dressing was applied. Patient was taken to the recovery room in stable condition.

No immediate complications were encountered.

The staff member was present and scrubbed for the entire procedure.

Chapter 54
Hammer Toe Correction

Bernard H. Sagherian, M.D.

COMMON INDICATIONS
- Hammer toe deformity with or without metatarsophalangeal joint subluxation

POSSIBLE COMPLICATIONS
- Recurrent deformity
- Pain
- Toe angulation
- Flexion deformity at the distal interphalangeal (DIP) joint
- Toe swelling
- Digital nerve and vessel injuries
- Infection

ESSENTIAL STEPS
1. Preoperative assessment (history, physical examination, radiographs)
2. Elliptical incisions over the dorsum of the proximal interphalangeal (PIP) joint with excision of the painful callus
3. Excision of adequate amount of bone to attain correction
4. Fixation of the arthrodesis site using 1.6 mm K-wire
5. Irrigation and closure of the wound without tension

OPERATIVE NOTE
Preoperative Diagnosis: Hammer toe deformity, second, third, or fourth

Procedure: Correction of hammer toe deformity by PIP joint fusion

Postoperative Diagnosis: Same

S. Saghieh et al. (eds.), *Operative Dictations in Orthopedic Surgery*,
DOI 10.1007/978-1-4614-7479-1_54,
© Springer Science+Business Media New York 2013

Indications: ___ years old patient with a painful fixed hammer toe deformity of the second toe (side) with a painful callus over the dorsum of the PIP joint.

Description of Operation: The operative site was checked and verified. IV antibiotics were administered and a tourniquet applied on the thigh. Under (type of anesthesia) and the patient in the supine position with a bump under the ipsilateral buttock the (side) lower extremity was prepped and draped.

An elliptical incision was made over the PIP joint excising the thickened skin. The incision was deepened and the extensor tendon was cut and the PIP joint capsule opened. Care was taken to protect the neurovascular bundle. The head of the proximal phalanx was identified. With a small micro-oscillating saw, the head was resected proximal to the condyles. Then the articular surface of the middle phalanx was also resected. Sharp edges were smoothened with a rasp. The resected edges were appositioned to ensure adequate correction of the deformity. A 1.6 mm K-wire was driven distally through the base of the middle phalanx, the bone edges are appositioned in the proper orientation, and the K-wire is driven proximally across the fusion site. The wound was irrigated and closed using 3-0 nylon sutures. The K-wire was cut and bent at the tip. A small dressing was applied. The patient tolerated the procedure well and was transferred to the post-anesthesia care unit in a stable condition.

Post-op regimen: weight-bearing as tolerated in a surgical shoe.

I was present for the entire procedure.

Chapter 55
Rheumatoid Foot Reconstruction

Geoffrey F. Haft, M.D.

COMMON INDICATIONS
- Pain unrelieved by nonoperative means
- Impending ulceration

POSSIBLE COMPLICATIONS
- Incisional problems
- Neurovascular problems
- Callus formation
- Gait instability
- First metatarsophalangeal nonunion

ESSENTIAL STEPS
1. Y-shaped incisions between second and third, fourth and fifth toes
2. Transection and resection of proximal end of proximal phalanx
3. Extensor tendon releases
4. Metatarsal head resections
5. Meticulous closure
6. Longitudinal medial incision over hallux MP joint
7. Metatarsal head prepared in conical shape
8. Gain access to proximal phalanx intramedullary canal
9. Reaming of proximal phalanx to create concavity
10. Positioning of MP joint in 15° of valgus, 25° plantar flexion
11. Internal fixation of hallux MP arthrodesis with 4.0 cancellous screw
12. Wound closure

S. Saghieh et al. (eds.), *Operative Dictations in Orthopedic Surgery*,
DOI 10.1007/978-1-4614-7479-1_55,
© Springer Science+Business Media New York 2013

OPERATIVE NOTE

Preoperative Diagnosis: Rheumatoid arthritis of foot

Procedure: Rheumatoid foot reconstruction

Postoperative Diagnosis: Same

Indications: __ yo woman with one of the indications above

Description of Operation: Pt was taken to the operating room and placed supine on the operating table. She was given 1 g of Ancef IV. After adequate regional/general anesthesia was obtained, the operative table was inclined in mild reverse Trendelenberg. The foot was positioned within inches of the end of the table. The calf was wrapped with an adequate amount of soft-rol and a tourniquet was placed. The leg was then prepped and draped in the standard sterile surgical fashion. The leg was exsanguinated with an Esmarch bandage and the tourniquet was raised to 100 mmHg greater than systolic pressure for a total of __ minutes.

Meticulous atraumatic technique was used throughout the case to protect the skin and soft tissues. A direct medial incision was used for the hallux and two Y-shaped longitudinal incisions were used for the lesser toes. The lesser toes were approached first using Y-shaped incisions in the web space between the second and third toes followed by the fourth and fifth toes. Starting with the second toe, thick flaps were developed by sharp dissection down to bone with the neurovascular bundle remaining in the plantar flap. The periosteum was stripped from the MP to the level of planned proximal phalanx transection. Bony excision was facilitated by removing as much investing soft tissue as possible. The proximal phalanx was stabilized with a towel clip and a small oscillating saw was used to cut across the diaphysis. The remaining soft tissue attachments were sharply released and the bone fragment delivered from the wound. The extensor tendon was then identified, isolated, and released. An identical procedure was then performed on the third through fifth toes, resecting slightly less of the proximal phalanx on each successive toe. Next, the metatarsal head resections were performed. The metatarsal heads were exposed by retraction of the capsule and excision of the pannus. A Carroll elevator was placed just proximal to the metatarsal condyle to shield soft tissue and establish the plantar level of bony transection. A small oscillating saw was used to excise the head just proximal to the dorsal articular edge, beveled 35° to the metatarsal shaft. All bony spikes were sharply excised. Each metatarsal head was excised in an identical manner. The fifth metatarsal was smoothed laterally to minimize risk of skin irritation. At the completion of the metatarsal head resections, there was 1–2 cm of space between the metatarsals and phalanges. Extreme care and precision was used in closing the syndactylization incisions. The flaps were gently closed using 4.0 nylon suture starting at the apex of the V and extended in a side-to-side manner from the plantar aspect around to the dorsum.

Next, attention was turned to arthrodesis of the first MP joint using a modification of McKeever's cup and cone technique. A 4 cm longitudinal incision was made on the medial border of the first MP joint. The dorsal and plantar nerves were identified and retracted, and the incision was deepened sharply, directly to bone. The metatarsal head and the most proximal aspect of the phalanx were exposed subperiosteally. The metatarsal head was then prepared to be shaped into a cone. A small oscillating saw was used to roughly define the cone's shape. The superolateral cortex was protected for eventual screw fixation. The metatarsal cone was finished by hand with the Marin reamer. Next, the proximal phalanx was cleared of soft tissues at its proximal end. A ¼ in. drill was used to establish access to the intramedullary canal. The surrounding cartilage was removed with a rongeur and the cup was excavated with a Marin reamer. The cup of proximal phalanx was then opposed to the metatarsal cone. Some adjustment was made around the base of the cone to establish close contact. The toe was positioned in approximately 15° of valgus and 25° of dorsiflexion and fixed provisionally with two parallel 0.035 in. K wires. Hallux position was reassessed to ensure that the pulp of the hallux was parallel or slightly dorsiflexed from the sole of the foot. The hallux lied within 5 mm of the second toe without touching it. Permanent fixation was achieved with a 4.0 cancellous screw placed from the medial cortex of the proximal phalanx base to the lateral cortex of the metatarsal neck. The position was reassessed and felt to be appropriate. The capsule of the first MP joint was closed with 2.0 absorbable braided suture and the skin was closed with a running 4.0 nylon suture. A nonadherent dressing with a single 4 × 4 gauze was placed over each wound and the forefoot wrapped with 2 in. gauze wrap. The wrap was passed around the pairs of syndactylized toes to hold them in slight plantar flexion. The entire foot was then protected in a compressive Robert Jones dressing.

The tourniquet was let down. The patient was awakened from anesthesia and sent to the recovery room in stable condition. Dr. _____ was present and scrubbed throughout the procedure.

Chapter 56

Repair of Acute Achilles Tendon Rupture

Bernard H. Sagherian, M.D.

COMMON INDICATIONS
- Complete rupture of the Achilles tendon

POSSIBLE COMPLICATIONS
- Re-rupture skin
- Wound necrosis
- Infection
- Sural nerve injury

ESSENTIAL STEPS
1. Preoperative assessment (history, physical examination, MRI)
2. Longitudinal incision medial to the Achilles tendon
3. Debridement of the tendon edges
4. Suture tendon
5. Closure of the peritenon
6. Irrigation, and wound closure without tension
7. Below-knee cast with the ankle in gravity equines

OPERATIVE NOTE
Preoperative Diagnosis: Achilles tendon rupture
Procedure: Repair of Achilles tendon rupture
Postoperative Diagnosis: Same
Indications: ___ years old patient with ruptured Achilles tendon (side)

S. Saghieh et al. (eds.), *Operative Dictations in Orthopedic Surgery,*
DOI 10.1007/978-1-4614-7479-1_56,
© Springer Science+Business Media New York 2013

Description of Operation: The operative site was checked and verified in the preoperative holding area. IV antibiotics were administered and a tourniquet applied on the thigh. Under (type of anesthesia) and the patient in the prone position, the (side) lower extremity was prepped and draped.

A 12 cm longitudinal skin incision was made on the medial border of the ruptured Achilles tendon starting distally at the tendinous insertion.

The incision was deepened through the subcutaneous tissue until the peritenon was reached and incised longitudinally in the direction of the skin incision. The ruptured Achilles tendon was identified. The hematoma was cleared using extensive irrigation. Debridement of the tendon edges was performed. The rupture was repaired using a double suture technique with nonabsorbable number 2 sutures. The repair was reenforced with interrupted absorbable vicryl 0 sutures. The peritenon was closed. The repair was checked by performing a Thompson's test and found to be excellent.

The tourniquet was deflated. The wound was thoroughly irrigated and closed using interrupted 3.0 nylon sutures.

Dressing was applied. The patient tolerated the procedure well and was transferred to the post-anesthesia care unit in stable condition.

Dr. _____ was present and scrubbed throughout the entire case.

Postop regimen: Application of below-knee cast with the ankle at gravity equines.

Increase in ankle dorsiflexion gradually over 6 weeks.

Chapter 57
Ankle Fusion

Michael J. Huang, M.D.

COMMON INDICATIONS
- Painful Arthritis

POSSIBLE COMPLICATIONS
- Neurologic damage
- Vascular damage
- Nonunion
- Infection
- Wound dehiscence
- Thromboembolic disease

ESSENTIAL STEPS
1. Lateral incision
2. Transfibular osteotomy
3. Removal of cartilage and subchondral bone in ankle joint
4. Possible medial arthrotomy to access medial aspect of joint
5. Alignment of joint
6. Screw and/or hardware placement
7. Irrigation
8. Packing of bone graft
9. Closure
10. Splint

OPERATIVE NOTE
Preoperative Diagnosis: End-stage ankle arthritis
Procedure: Ankle fusion Rt/Lt

S. Saghieh et al. (eds.), *Operative Dictations in Orthopedic Surgery*,
DOI 10.1007/978-1-4614-7479-1_57,
© Springer Science+Business Media New York 2013

Postoperative Diagnosis: Same

Indications: End-stage ankle arthritis, failed conservative therapy

Description of Operation: The patient was brought to the operating room after a fem-popliteal block was given. The lower extremity was prepped and draped in the usual sterile fashion. Tourniquet was applied and inflated to 350 mmHg.

Through a lateral approach, the distal 5 cm of the fibula was resected. The ankle joint was explored and the articular cartilage curetted on both sides of the joint. An anterior medial arthrotomy was performed. Resection of the articular cartilage was completed from this side as well. Any surface irregularity in the subchondral bone was adjusted with the use of straight osteotome. The talus and the tibial plafond surfaces were checked to be parallel and perpendicular to the axis of the tibia in both planes. The ankle joint was then fixed with two k-wires in neutral position in the frontal and sagittal plane, approximately 10° of external rotation, neutral to slight valgus of the heel, and posterior positioning of the talus.

The guide wires were then inserted from posterior superior to anterior inferior in a crossing pattern. Drilling was then performed followed by tapping and insertion of the appropriate length 7 mm cannulated, half-threaded screws. Position was checked by fluoroscopy.

The resected fibula was morcelized and the bone chips used as bone graft around the fusion.

We then irrigated and closed in a layered fashion; the subcutaneous tissue was closed with 2-0 Vicryl, and the skin with 3-0 nylon.

A sterile dressing was applied on the foot as well as a short leg splint. The tourniquet was deflated and the patient was transferred to the recovery room in good conditions.

Dr. ___ was present and scrubbed for the entire case.

Chapter 58

Subtalar Fusion

John-Erik Bell, M.D., M.S.

COMMON INDICATIONS
- Subtalar arthrosis secondary to trauma
- Rheumatoid arthritis
- Coalition
- Subtalar instability

POSSIBLE COMPLICATIONS
- Nonunion
- Malunion
- Infection

ESSENTIAL STEPS
1. Positioning—place bump under hip to internally rotate, place calf tourniquet
2. Visualization, cartilage removal of all facets
3. Correct any varus/valgus deformity by removing a wedge—goal is 5–10° of valgus
4. Feathering/drilling
5. Bone grafting (auto, allo, or bone substitute)
6. Fixation—must cross posterior facet, use washer, 7.3 cannulated screw

OPERATIVE NOTE
Preoperative Diagnosis: Isolated subtalar arthritis
Procedure: Subtalar fusion
Postoperative Diagnosis: Same
Description of Operation: The patient was identified and the site of surgery confirmed. Anesthesia was induced. Prophylactic IV antibiotics were administered. The patient was placed supine on a radiolucent operating table, a padded calf tourniquet was placed,

S. Saghieh et al. (eds.), *Operative Dictations in Orthopedic Surgery*,
DOI 10.1007/978-1-4614-7479-1_58,
© Springer Science+Business Media New York 2013

the foot was shaved, a bump was placed under the ipsilateral hip, and all bony prominences were padded. The patient was then prepped and draped. Tourniquet was inflated to 300 mmHg.

An incision was made from the tip of the fibula to the base of the fourth metatarsal and carried to the level of the fascia taking care to protect the sural nerve. The fascia was then incised over the extensor digitorum brevis (EDB). The EDB was then elevated distally to the calcaneocuboid joint. The fat pad of the sinus tarsi was then removed exposing the posterior facet of the subtalar joint. The joint was then opened with a lamina spreader. A sharp osteotome was used to remove all articular cartilage from the posterior and middle facets. The bony surfaces were then drilled to promote bleeding and fusion with a 2.5 drill bit. Alignment was assessed and found to be in acceptable valgus (5–10°).

Bone allograft was then packed into the fusion site and the sinus tarsi. A 2.8 mm threaded guide wire was then introduced from the posteroinferior surface of the calcaneal tuberosity (just above the weight-bearing surface) across the posterior facet into the junction of the talar neck and body. The wire was then over-drilled, tapped, and a 7.3 mm partially threaded screw placed over a washer. Screw length and position were checked with fluoroscopy. Tourniquet was deflated and hemostasis achieved.

The wound was thoroughly irrigated, the fascia closed with 2-0 vicryl, and the skin with nylon suture. Dressing was applied and the foot was placed in a plaster splint in neutral dorsiflexion.

The patient was awakened from anesthesia and sent to the recovery room in stable condition.

Chapter 59

Triple Arthrodesis: Fusion of the Subtalar, Calcaneocuboid, and Talonavicular Joints

Karim Masrouha, M.D.

COMMON INDICATIONS
- Correction of fixed hindfoot deformities
- Control of progressive hindfoot deformities
- Painful arthritis

POSSIBLE COMPLICATIONS
- Wound healing problems/infection
- Nonunion
- Malunion
- DVT

ESSENTIAL STEPS
1. Lateral skin incision
2. Expose and denude cartilage of the talocalcaneal joint
3. Expose and denude cartilage of the calcaneocuboid joint
4. Medial skin incision
5. Expose and denude cartilage of the talonavicular joint
6. Reduction of the joints in good position
7. Fixation of the talocalcaneal joint
8. Fixation of the talonavicular joint
9. Fixation of the calcaneocuboid
10. Closure

OPERATIVE NOTE
Preoperative Diagnosis: Painful stiff subtalar joint, L/R
Procedure: Triple arthrodesis, left/ right foot

S. Saghieh et al. (eds.), *Operative Dictations in Orthopedic Surgery*,
DOI 10.1007/978-1-4614-7479-1_59,
© Springer Science+Business Media New York 2013

Postoperative Diagnosis: Same

Indications: The patient has a painful and stiff subtalar joint after sustaining an intraarticular subtalar fracture 3 years ago. The patient has failed conservative treatment, and after a long discussion of surgical options the patient wished to proceed with triple arthrodesis.

Description of Operation: The patient and surgical site were identified marked.

The patients underwent anesthesia per the anesthesia team. The patient was positioned in the supine position with a sand bag beneath the R/L buttock. All bony prominences were well padded. A tourniquet was placed over the proximal thigh. The leg was then prepped and draped in the standard sterile fashion. The extremity was exsanguinated and the tourniquet was inflated to 300 mmHg.

A straight lateral incision was performed running from 1 cm inferior to the tip of the lateral malleolus to the base of fourth metatarsal distally. The incision was deepened through the subcutaneous tissue; the sheath of the peroneal tendon was incised in its most anterior portion; the peroneal tendons and the sural nerve were retracted posteriorly.

The extensor digitorum brevis and extensor hallucis brevis were dissected off the sinus tarsi that were cleared from soft tissues. The subtalar joint was identified. The cartilage was denuded from the posterior, middle, and anterior facets of the subtalar joint using osteotomes and small rongeur. A laminar spreader was introduced to aid in this process. The extensor digitorum brevis belly was followed from proximal to distal to identify the calcaneocuboid joint. The capsule was cleared from soft tissue attachments and was opened to expose the joint.

The articular cartilage was removed from both sides of the joint using small osteotomes and curets.

A 5 cm medial longitudinal skin incision was then performed in line and medial to the tibialis anterior tendon. Sharp dissection was carried down through the tibialis anterior tendon sheath. The talonavicular joint was exposed at this level. The articular cartilage was denuded from both sides of the joint with an osteotome and curet.

The three joints were reduced and hold in an anatomical plantigrade position with the hindfoot in 8–10° of valgus and the talonavicular and calcaneocuboid joints in proper sagittal and axial planes as well as in proper rotation.

A threaded guidepin was passed from the corner of the heel (approximately 1 cm lateral to the midline of the tuberosity of the calcaneus near the junction of the heel pad and the skin covering the hindfoot) to the superior cortex of the talar neck (just distal to the body–neck junction).

This was over-drilled and tapped. Allograft was packed into the subtalar joint before the insertion of the cannulated 7 mm partially threaded -- mm length screw.

Next, a separate stab incision was utilized to pass a threaded guidepin from medial plantar aspect of the navicular to lateral and dorsal talus under fluoroscopic guidance.

This was measured at -- mm and the guidepin was over-drilled and then a 7 mm/-- long partially threaded screw was introduced and seated into position. Bone graft was also packed into this joint with a bone tamp.

Lastly, another threaded guide pin was passed from the cuboid to the calcaneus through a separate stab incision between the base of the fourth and fifth metatarsals.

It was sized and overdrilled. A -- mm cannulated screw was inserted to complete the fusion. Once again, bone was packed into this joint with allograft and a bone tamp and mallet.

Next, copious irrigation with normal saline was performed. Fluoroscopic check of reduction as well as screw lengths was checked and found to be excellent. The wounds were then closed in two layers; the subcutaneous tissue with 2-0 Vicryl, and the skin with 3-0 nylon in a horizontal mattress fashion. The foot was then dressed with Adaptic, 4×4 gauze, sterile soft roll, and then a U splint was applied and the foot was held in position until the splint had hardened.

The patient was awakened and transferred to the PACU in stable condition.

No intra-operative complications.

Staff was present and scrubbed for the entire procedure.

Chapter 60
Total Ankle Replacement

Said Saghieh, M.D.

COMMON INDICATIONS
- Inflammatory or degenerative arthritis of the ankle joint

POSSIBLE COMPLICATIONS
- Infection
- Loosening
- Pain
- Instability

ESSENTIAL STEPS
1. Careful preoperative clinical and radiographic assessment
2. Ankle distractor application on the medial side
3. Anterior longitudinal incision
4. Osteotomies: tibia and talus
5. Implants
6. Lateral incision for syndesmosis
7. Closure

OPERATIVE NOTE
Preoperative Diagnosis: Arthritis, ankle
Procedure: Total ankle replacement
Postoperative Diagnosis: Same
Indications: ___ year-old male/female who has been complaining of ankle pain of several months duration resistant to conservative treatment.
Description of Operation: The patient and the surgical site were identified and marked in the preholding area. The patient underwent anesthesia per the anesthesia team.

S. Saghieh et al. (eds.), *Operative Dictations in Orthopedic Surgery*,
DOI 10.1007/978-1-4614-7479-1_60,

The patient was placed supine with a sandbag under the affected side. A thigh tourniquet was applied. The lower extremity was prepped and draped in the usual manner.

A bone distractor was placed on the medial side and used to distract the ankle by 5 mm and to correct any deformity.

Next, the tourniquet was inflated to 350 mmHg. A 10 cm longitudinal anterior incision was performed and deepened between the extensor hallucis longus and the anterior tibial tendons. The superficial peroneal nerve was retracted laterally.

The anterior capsule was incised longitudinally and subperiosteal dissection was carried to expose the distal tibia. Osteophytes were removed from the anterior lip of the tibia plafond.

A longitudinal deep incision was made along the anterior border of the distal fibula and the anterior tibiofibular ligament was excised and the syndesmosis was mobilized.

The jig alignment guide was centered just distal to the tibial tubercle in line with the axis of the tibia. The cutting block was centered over the ankle joint and the tibia and the talus osteotomies performed.

Tibial and talar trial components were inserted and inspected for range of motion and stability.

Appropriate implants were then cemented on both sides and the ankle distractor was removed.

Through the lateral incision, the tibiofibular syndesmosis was decorticated and morselized bone that has been resected from the tibia and talus was placed into this interval. The syndesmosis was secured by two screws.

After thorough irrigation, the wounds were closed in a routine-layered manner.

Sterile dressing and compression dressing were applied as well as a posterior splint. Tourniquet was deflated.

No intraoperative complications.

Staff was present and scrubbed for entire procedure.

Chapter 61
Tarsal Coalition Resection

Karim Masrouha, M.D.

COMMON INDICATIONS
- Persistent pain following conservative treatment of a tarsal coalition

POSSIBLE COMPLICATIONS
- Persistent pain
- Injury to the sural nerve
- Infection

There are multiple types of tarsal coalitions. Operative procedures for resection of the two most common types are described below.

CALCANEONAVICULAR COALITION RESECTION
Essential Steps
1. Tourniquet placement
2. Lateral skin incision
3. Extensor digitorum brevis (EDB) muscle reflected from calcaneus
4. Identification and resection of coalition
5. Interposition of EDB origin and surrounding fat tissue into coalition resection site
6. Irrigation and wound closure
7. Application of non-weight-bearing short leg cast

OPERATIVE NOTE
Preoperative Diagnosis: Calcaneonavicular coalition
Procedure: Resection of calcaneonavicular coalition
Postoperative Diagnosis: Same

S. Saghieh et al. (eds.), *Operative Dictations in Orthopedic Surgery*,
DOI 10.1007/978-1-4614-7479-1_61,
© Springer Science+Business Media New York 2013

Indications: __ years old male/female with persistent foot pain and decreased subtalar range of motion. On physical examination, the patient has a flatfoot deformity and the heel remains in a valgus position when the patient stands on tiptoes. The patient also has pain with passive inversion of the hindfoot. Plain radiographs/CT/MRI shows evidence of calcaneonavicular coalition. The patient continued to have pain despite treatment in a short leg walking cast for 2–4 weeks.

Description of Operation: The patient and surgical site were identified and marked. The patient underwent anesthesia per the anesthesia team. The patient was placed in the supine position on the operating table and all pressure points were padded. A tourniquet was placed on the thigh over a soft roll. Intravenous antibiotics were administered. The left/right lower extremity was prepped and draped in the standard sterile fashion. The extremity was exsanguinated and the tourniquet was inflated to 300 mmHg.

An oblique incision was made from near the heel to the head of the talus on the lateral aspect of the foot. Care was taken to protect branches of the sural nerve (lateral dorsal cutaneous nerve). The EDB muscle was identified and reflected from its origin on the calcaneus, providing access to the calcaneonavicular joint. The coalition was then identified and resected with a small osteotome and rongeur. Increased motion between the calcaneus and navicular was then confirmed. A Bunnell suture was passed through the origin of the EDB muscle. Keith needles were used to pass the sutures through the area of the coalition to the medial aspect of the midfoot. The EDB muscle and some surrounding fat tissue were pulled into the area of the coalition resection and the sutures were secured over a cotton-padded button on the medial midfoot. The tourniquet was released and hemostasis was obtained. The wound was irrigated and closed in two layers; subcutaneous tissue with vicryl 2.0 and skin with monocryl 4.0 in subcuticular fashion. A short leg cast was applied with the foot in neutral position.

The patient was then awakened and transferred to the PACU in stable condition.

No intra-operative complications.

Staff was present and scrubbed for the entire procedure.

TALOCALCANEAL COALITION RESECTION
Essential Steps
1. Tourniquet placement
2. Prep and drape lower abdomen/suprapubic area for fat graft harvest

3. Incision over sustentaculum tali
4. Identification and retraction of abductor hallucis longus
5. Division of flexor retinaculum
6. Identification and retraction of flexor digitorum longus, posterior tibial artery, tibial nerve, flexor hallucis longus, posterior tibialis tendon
7. Periosteum opening
8. Coalition resection
9. Fat graft interposition
10. Periosteum closure

OPERATIVE NOTE

Preoperative Diagnosis: Talocalcaneal coalition
Procedure: Resection of talocalcaneal coalition
Postoperative Diagnosis: Same
Indications: __ years old male/female with persistent foot pain and decreased subtalar range of motion. On physical exam, the patient has a flatfoot deformity and the heel remains in a valgus position when the patient stands on tiptoes. The patient also has pain with passive inversion of the hindfoot. Plain films/CT shows evidence of talocalcaneal coalition. The patient continued to have pain despite treatment in a short leg walking cast for 2–4 weeks.
Description of Operation: The patient and surgical site were identified and marked. The patient underwent anesthesia as per the anesthesia team. The patient was placed in the supine position on the operating table and all pressure points were padded. Intravenous antibiotics were administered. A tourniquet was placed on the thigh over a soft roll. The left/right lower extremity was prepped and draped in the standard sterile fashion. The extremity was exsanguinated and the tourniquet was inflated to 300 mmHg.

A curvilinear incision was made over the sustentaculum tali. The flexor retinaculum was divided over the sustentaculum tali. Then the neurovascular bundle (posterior tibial artery and tibial nerve) was retracted plantarward and the flexor digitorum longus and posterior tibialis tendons were retracted dorsally. The flexor hallucis longus was identified and retracted plantarward. The periosteum was reflected off of the sustentaculum tali. The anterior and posterior margins of the coalition were identified with needles and the coalition was then resected using a high speed burr.

The resection was considered complete when a rim of articular cartilage of the middle facet became visible and the subtalar joint was mobile.

A 2 cm incision was made in the lower abdomen. A small amount of subcutaneous fat was removed. Hemostasis was obtained and the abdominal wound was closed with a 3-0 monocryl subcuticular suture.

The fat graft was placed in the area of the talonavicular coalition resection. The periosteum was closed using vicryl 2.0. The tourniquet was let down and hemostasis was obtained. The wound was closed in two layers; subcutaneous tissue with vicryl 3.0 and skin with monocryl 4.0 in subcuticular fashion. A short leg non-weight-bearing cast was applied with the foot in neutral position.

The patient was then awakened and transferred to the PACU in stable condition.

No intra-operative complications.

Staff was present and scrubbed for the entire procedure.

Chapter 62
Lateral Ankle Ligament Reconstruction: Brostrom Type

Karim Masrouha, M.D.

COMMON INDICATIONS
- Recurrent ankle sprain
- Chronic instability

POSSIBLE COMPLICATIONS
- Infection
- Thromboembolism
- Injury to the superficial peroneal nerve and/or sural nerve
- Rupture of the repair or stretching out of the ligament
- Stiffness

ESSENTIAL STEPS
1. Preoperative assessment and planning (history, physical examination, evaluation of radiographs)
2. Incision of skin and dissection
3. Incision of extensor retinaculum
4. Identification of peroneal tendon sheath and tendons
5. Incision of the capsule around the fibula and identification of the ligamentous thickenings
6. Decortication of the fibular edges
7. Insertion of suture anchors on fibula
8. Tensioning of the ligaments and tying to the sutures
9. Repair of the fibular periosteum over ligaments
10. Closure of capsular tissues over ligaments

S. Saghieh et al. (eds.), *Operative Dictations in Orthopedic Surgery*,
DOI 10.1007/978-1-4614-7479-1_62,
© Springer Science+Business Media New York 2013

11. Reinforcement of repair with repair of the extensor retinaculum
12. Irrigation and closure
13. Cast/splint placement

OPERATIVE NOTE

Preoperative Diagnosis: Chronic left/right lateral ankle instability

Procedure: Brostrom reconstruction of the L/R lateral ankle ligaments

Postoperative Diagnosis: Same

Indications: __ year old male/female with recurrent left/right ankle sprains and symptoms of chronic instability. The patient has failed conservative treatment with bracing and, after explaining the risks and benefits of this procedure, has elected to proceed with operative management.

Description of Operation: The patient and surgical site were identified and marked. The patient underwent anesthesia per the anesthesia team. The patient was placed in the supine position on the operating table and all pressure points were padded. A tourniquet was placed on the thigh over a soft-roll. The left/right lower extremity was then prepped and draped in the standard sterile fashion. The extremity was exsanguinated and the tourniquet was inflated to 300 mmHg. Intravenous antibiotics were administered.

A longitudinal incision was made along the posterior edge of the fibula crossing the fibula inferiorly and towards the area of the talar neck. Sharp and blunt dissection was used to proceed through all of the subcutaneous tissues. The anterior edge of the extensor retinaculum was identified and was incised. Next, the peroneal tendon sheath was identified and opened longitudinally and the tendons were inspected. (There were no abnormalities of the peroneal tendons.) The joint capsule was identified and incised in its full thickness around the fibula. The thickenings representing the insertions of the calcaneofibular ligament as well as the talofibular ligaments were identified. The bony edges of the fibula were decorticated. Anchor sutures were then implanted into the fibula at the insertion of the calcaneofibular ligament and then along the insertion of the anterior talofibular ligament. All three of the lateral ligaments, having previously been identified and dissected off as one layer, were then pulled proximally and attached to the anchor sutures. The periosteum of the fibula was then brought over these ligaments and repaired using nonabsorbable suture. Capsular tissues were then repaired and further imbricated with the ligaments at this point. The foot was held in slight dorsiflexion and neutral eversion for the whole repair process.

The extensor retinaculum was then rotated over the repair and sutured to the anterior lateral edge of the fibula to further reinforce the repair. The peroneal sheath was repaired using 2.0 vicryl suture. The wound was copiously irrigated and the tourniquet was released. Hemostasis was secured. The subcutaneous tissues were closed with vicryl 3.0, and the skin closed with staples. The wound was dressed and the patient was placed in a short leg cast with the foot in slight dorsiflexion and eversion.

The patient was then awakened and transferred to the PACU in stable condition.

No intra-operative complications.

Staff was present and scrubbed for entire procedure.

Postoperative regimen: Application of a short leg cast. Strict elevation of the knee above the heart for 5 days. Non-weightbearing for 2 weeks followed by progressive weightbearing, with physical therapy including proprioception and muscle strengthening exercises started at 6 weeks postoperatively.

Chapter 63

Distal Tibia Fracture: Nonbridging Hybrid External Fixator

Said Saghieh, M.D.

COMMON INDICATIONS
- Extra-articular pillon fractures
- Intra-articular pillon fractures without gross comminution of the articular surface
- Pillon fractures with soft tissue injury

POSSIBLE COMPLICATIONS
- Failure of reduction
- Malunion
- Nonunion
- Pin site infection
- DVT

ESSENTIAL STEPS
1. Careful preoperative assessment and planning
2. ORIF of tibial plafond with screws
3. Application of the ring on the distal part of the fracture
4. Application of the half pins on the proximal part of the fracture
5. Reduction of the main fracture

OPERATIVE NOTE
Preoperative Diagnosis: Intra-articular pillon fracture with T-shaped fracture line of the ankle
Procedure: Limited internal fixation of pillon fracture with application of nonbridging hybrid fixator
Postoperative Diagnosis: Same

S. Saghieh et al. (eds.), *Operative Dictations in Orthopedic Surgery*,
DOI 10.1007/978-1-4614-7479-1_63,
© Springer Science+Business Media New York 2013

Indications: ___ year-old male/female who sustained a comminuted intra-articular fracture of the R/L ankle with skin contusion.

Description of Operation: The patient and operative site were identified and marked by the surgeon in the preoperative holding area. Then the patient was brought to the operating room and was placed supine on the operative table. He/she was given general anesthesia. IV antibiotics (1 g of Ancef) were administered.

All bony prominences were well padded. A padded sand bag was placed under the hip to rotate the patella into the AP plane.

The fracture was again evaluated with fluoroscopy marking the intra-articular component, the main fracture line, and the proximal extent of the fracture.

With manual traction, we achieved reduction of the intra-articular part. This was fixed with two 4 mm cannulated screws introduced over guide wires that were measured, drilled, and tapped over (length: --- and --- mm).

The hybrid frame was selected with an appropriate diameter of the distal ring to allow clearance of the surrounding soft tissue (150 mm).

The ring was placed over the distal fragment. Two pairs of wire clamps were placed over the ring. The first two 2 mm wires were inserted from posteromedial (but anterior to the post-tibialis tendon) to anterolateral paying attention to hammer them once they exit the second cortex to minimize the risk of anterior neurovascular bundle injury. The next pair of wires was inserted from posterolateral side transfixing the distal fibula and exiting through the anteromedial aspect of the tibia. The angle between these two pairs of wires was 60°. All these wires were parallel to the joint line in both planes. The wires were tensioned to 1,200 N with the appropriate tensioning device. Wire clamp screws were tightened over with 5 mm Allen wrench. Wires were then bent and cut.

The fracture was reduced by manipulation of the ring and the limb. The straight fixator was then aligned parallel to the long axis of the tibia and attached to the ring.

The fixator body was mounted half-opened to allow later distraction or compression. The proximal clamp was used as a template to apply three 6 mm conical half pins through its first, third and fifth holes. A 4.8 mm drill bit was used first to drill holes perpendicular to the anteromedial face of the tibial shaft in both frontal and sagittal planes. The adequate length of the half pins was measured and the appropriate three half pins applied (130/30 mm). The clamp was tightened over the pins.

The reduction was confirmed again by fluoroscopy. Axial alignment in both planes and correct rotation were obtained before tightening the central body locking nut and the connecting cam.

A reinforcement bar was used to increase the stiffness of the fixation (delta configuration).

A sterile dressing was applied over the leg.

There was no intraoperative complication.

Staff was present and scrubbed for entire procedure.

Chapter 64
Ankle Fracture: Open Reduction and Internal Fixation

Robert Frangie

COMMON INDICATIONS
- Bimalleolar ankle fracture

POSSIBLE COMPLICATIONS
- Loss of reduction
- Malunion
- Nonunion
- Wound infection
- Stiffness
- Ankle arthrosis

ESSENTIAL STEPS
Fixation of Lateral Malleolus
1. Expose the lateral malleolus and the distal fibular shaft through a posterolateral longitudinal incision.
2. Protect the superficial peroneal nerve.
3. Anatomical reduction and maintenance of fibular length are necessary.
4. Place a lag screw inserted from anterior to posterior across the fracture to establish compression.
5. A 1/3 tubular plate is placed on the posterolateral or direct lateral aspect of the fibula with 2–3 fixation points proximal and distal to the fracture.

Fixation of Medial Malleolus
1. Make an anteromedial incision beginning 1 cm proximal to the fracture line, extending distally and slightly posteriorly ending 2 cm distal to the tip of the medial malleolus.

S. Saghieh et al. (eds.), *Operative Dictations in Orthopedic Surgery*,
DOI 10.1007/978-1-4614-7479-1_64,
© Springer Science+Business Media New York 2013

2. Carefully reflect the skin flaps with the underlying subcutaneous tissue, protecting the saphenous nerve and greater saphenous vein.

3. Inspect the medial gutter of the ankle joint to assess the talus for osteochondral injuries.

4. Remove any interposed loose fragments or periosteum from between the fracture surfaces with a curet or periosteal elevator.

5. Reduce the medial malleolus and evaluate the reduction at the articular surface through the incision.

6. Pin the medial malleolus fragment with 0.045 in. k-wires in a parallel fashion.

7. Check the fracture reduction with fluoroscopy.

8. Drill and place a 4.0 mm partially threaded malleolar screw in the posterior portion of the fragment perpendicular to the fracture line.

9. Remove one of the k-wires then drill and place a second 4.0 partially threaded malleolar screw in the anterior portion of the fragment parallel to the first screw.

OPERATIVE NOTE

Preoperative Diagnosis: Right/left ankle bimalleolar fracture

Procedure: Open reduction and internal fixation of right/left ankle bimalleolar fracture

Postoperative Diagnosis: Same

Indication: … years old male/female with right/left ankle bimalleolar fracture post trauma

Description of Operation: The patient was identified in the preoperative holding and the correct extremity confirmed. He was brought into the operating room and placed supine on the operating table. General anesthesia was delivered and IV antibiotics given. A tourniquet was applied over the proximal thigh. The right/left lower extremity was prepped and draped in the sterile usual manner. Tourniquet was inflated to 350 mmHg. An 8 cm longitudinal incision was made from the tip of the lateral malleolus extending proximally over the posterolateral aspect of the fibula. Sharp dissection was performed down to bone where the fracture hematoma and elevated periosteum were encountered. The superficial peroneal was protected by the anterior reflection of the peronei muscles. The fracture ends of the fibula were identified and curetted without stripping the fracture ends. The soft tissues immediately adjacent to the fracture line were elevated approximately 2 mm to clearly identify the fracture plane. Anatomic reduction of the fibula was obtained by distraction, and reversing the mechanism of injury. The reduction was then maintained with pointed tenaculums compressing perpendicular to the fracture line. The projected path of an anterior to posterior interfragmentary lag screw oriented perpendicular to the fracture line (parallel to the pointed reduction tenaculums) was planned. A 3.5 drill was used to create the gliding hole and the second cortex was drilled with a 2.7 drill. A 3.5 mm fully threaded cortical screw was then placed in to lag the fragment together. A ___ hole 1/3 tubular neutralization plate was placed across the fracture over the periosteum. Two (or three) 3.5 mm fully threaded cortical screws were placed into the proximal fragment obtaining bicortical purchase. The distal fragment was secured with two fully threaded cancellous screws. Fluoroscopy was used to confirm extra-articular placement of these screws.

A 3 cm incision was then made along the anteromedial aspect of the medial malleolus. Blunt dissection allowed identification of the saphanous nerve and greater saphanous vein. These structures were retracted and sharp dissection was performed to the anterior margin of the fracture site. The fracture fragments were identified visually and existing hematoma was removed. The fracture site was curetted and irrigated. Interposed torn periosteum was removed from the fracture site. The talus articular surface was inspected for lesions and none were present. The distal fragment was then manipulated with the aid of a reduction awl. Anatomic reduction was obtained while visualizing both the outer cortex and the articular surface. Provisional reduction was maintained with two 0.045 in. k-wires inserted from the tip of the medial malleolus directed proximal and lateral in a parallel fashion. Fluoroscopy was used to confirm the reduction. A 2.7 mm drill was then used to drill the posterior screw path (parallel to the k-wires). A 4.0 mm partially threaded cancellous screw (45 mm in length) was then inserted. One of the k-wires was removed and second screw was placed in a similar fashion in the anterior portion of the fragment parallel to the first screw.

Final fluoroscopic images were obtained and an assessment of the syndesmosis was performed fluoroscopically. After confirming an anatomic reduction of the ankle mortise without evidence of instability, the wounds were irrigated with normal saline. The fascial tissues were closed in an interrupted fashion with vicryl 2.0 to cover the hardware. The skin was then closed in a tension-free manner with 3-0 nylon suture in a vertical mattress fashion. Bactigras was placed over both incisions and the foot was then wrapped with sterile soft roll. A plaster splint was applied to allow for postoperative swelling. Needle and sponge counts were correct and the patient was awakened from anesthesia.

Staff was present and scrubbed during the procedure.

Chapter 65

Lisfranc Open Reduction and Internal Fixation

Robert Frangie

COMMON INDICATIONS
- Lisfranc displaced fractures with or without dislocations
- Lisfranc's complex injuries

POSSIBLE COMPLICATIONS
- Persistent midfoot pain
- Nonunion
- Malunion
- Nerve or vessel damage
- Hardware complications or pain, infection, compartment syndrome

ESSENTIAL STEPS
1. Careful preoperative assessment (history, physical examination—evaluation of compartment syndrome, radiographs)
2. Use of any combination of three dorsal incisions depending upon locations of injury to expose fractures with protection of neurovascular and tendon structures
3. Anatomic reduction and provisional stabilization of midfoot under fluoroscopic guidance
4. ORIF with standard technique of midfoot: screw fixation of the medial midfoot and k-wire fixation for the lateral midfoot
5. Irrigation, debridement, and closure of incisions
6. Short leg splint application

S. Saghieh et al. (eds.), *Operative Dictations in Orthopedic Surgery*,
DOI 10.1007/978-1-4614-7479-1_65,
© Springer Science+Business Media New York 2013

OPERATIVE NOTE

Preoperative Diagnosis: Lisfranc displaced fracture dislocation

Procedure: ORIF Lisfranc fracture dislocation

Postoperative Diagnosis: Same

Indications: ___ yo male/female who sustained a longitudinal/axial load to the plantar flexed foot sustaining a complex Lisfranc fracture dislocation with displacement.

Description of Operation: The patient and surgical site were identified and marked. The patient underwent general endotracheal anesthesia. The patient was positioned supine on the operative table with all bony prominences padded. A tourniquet was placed on the thigh over a cotton-roll. IV antibiotics were administered.

Fluoroscopy was used to assess the stability of each column of the foot to plan the reduction and the stabilization. The injured lower extremity was then prepped and draped in the usual sterile fashion.

A dorsal 5 cm longitudinal incision was made just lateral to the EHL, extending from the navicular to the first metatarsal space. Careful sharp dissection with minimal soft tissue disruption was carried out through the soft tissues. The EHL was retracted medially and the dorsalis pedis artery and the deep peroneal nerve were retracted laterally. The capsule over the base of second metatarsal was incised and the articular surface of the middle cuneiform was identified. The first and second TMT joints were reduced checking for both rotational and angular alignment. Provisional stabilization was performed using the threaded guide wires. A second incision was made from the cuboid to the third web space distally. The superficial peroneal nerve was protected. The lateral border of the third metatarsal was reduced to the lateral border of the lateral cuneiform. A guide wire was used to fix the lateral column going from the fourth metatarsal to the cuboid. Reduction was checked again under fluoroscopy before overdrilling the guide wires and insertion of the appropriate 4 mm partially threaded cannulated screws.

Wounds were irrigated and closed with 2-vicryl and 3-0 nylon. Sterile dressings and a splint were applied.

Postop regimen: Application of a short leg cast. Strict elevation. Non-weight bearing for 3 months.

No intraoperative complications.

Staff was present and scrubbed for entire procedure.

Chapter 66

Talus Open Reduction and Internal Fixation

Geoffrey F. Haft, M.D.

COMMON INDICATIONS
- Any displaced talar neck fracture (Hawkins Type II, III, and IV)
- Any open fracture of the talus

POSSIBLE COMPLICATIONS
- Infection
- Skin necrosis
- Avascular necrosis
- Posttraumatic arthritis
- Neurovascular injury
- Malunion
- Nonunion

ESSENTIAL STEPS
Posterior Approach
1. Incision just lateral to Achilles tendon
2. Posterior process of talus identified between FHL and peroneus brevis
3. Closed reduction obtained with fluoroscopic guidance
4. Reduction held in place with two K-wires
5. Rigid fixation obtained with two parallel 4.0 mm cancellous screws
6. Screws placed perpendicular to fracture site
7. Position of screws checked on fluoro to ensure they don't violate talonavicular joint

S. Saghieh et al. (eds.), *Operative Dictations in Orthopedic Surgery*,
DOI 10.1007/978-1-4614-7479-1_66,
© Springer Science+Business Media New York 2013

Anteromedial Approach

1. Incision just medial to tibialis anterior tendon.
2. Care taken to protect saphenous vein and nerve.
3. Dissection carried down to talar neck.
4. If necessary to see fracture site, medial malleolus osteotomy performed.
5. Open reduction of fracture achieved.
6. Reduction held in place with two K-wires.
7. Reduction confirmed with fluoroscopy.
8. Rigid fixation obtained with two parallel 4.0 mm cancellous screws from nonarticular surface of talar neck.
9. Screws placed perpendicular to fracture site.
10. Position of screws checked on fluoro to ensure they don't violate surrounding joints.

OPERATIVE NOTE

Preoperative Diagnosis: Displaced talar neck fracture
Procedure: ORIF talus
Postoperative Diagnosis: Same
Indications: __ yo patient with displace talar neck fracture
Description of Operation: Pt was taken to the operating room and placed supine on the operating table. She was given 1 g of Ancef IV. After adequate regional/general anesthesia was obtained, the leg was wrapped with an adequate amount of soft-rol and a tourniquet was placed. The leg was then prepped and draped in the standard sterile surgical fashion. The leg was exsanguinated with an Esmarch bandage and the tourniquet was raised to 350 mmHg for a total of __ minutes.

For a Hawkins type II fracture, the posterolateral approach generally works well as the fracture can usually be reduced by closed means using fluoroscopic guidance. The patient was placed in the lateral decubitus position with the noninjured side down. An axillary roll was placed and all bony prominences and nerves were carefully padded. A 4 cm long incision was made just lateral to the Achilles tendon. Care was taken to protect the sural nerve, just anterior to the incision site. The posterior process of the talus was located between the flexor hallucis longus and peroneus brevis tendons. A closed reduction was performed by plantar flexing and abducting the forefoot under fluoroscopic guidance. A 2.0 mm K-wire was placed in the body of the talus to manipulate the fracture into an anatomic position. The reduction was checked fluoroscopically using lateral, Canale, and Broden's views. Next, two K-wires were driven from the nonarticular aspect of the talar body across the fracture site into the talar head to hold the reduction. The reduction was reassessed with fluoro. Next, rigid fixation was achieved by drilling, tapping, and placing two 4.0 mm parallel cancellous screws across the fracture site. Maximum compression was obtained by placing these screws perpendicular to the fracture plane. The threads extended across the fracture site, but not into the talonavicular joint. The wound was thoroughly irrigated with normal saline and closed with interrupted 4.0 nylon stitches in a vertical mattress fashion. The wound was dressed with non-stick gauze, 4 × 4's, and sterile soft roll. A posterior plaster splint was applied and wrapped with an Ace bandage.

Most Hawkins type III and IV fractures require open reduction. The most commonly used anteromedial approach is described. This approach is usually done in the supine position. A 4 cm longitudinal incision was made just medial to the tibialis anterior tendon. Care was taken to avoid the saphenous vein and nerve. The dissection was then carried down to the ankle joint capsule and the neck of the talus. In order to better visualize the talar neck, the dissection was carried more medial in a subcutaneous fashion, and a medial malleolus osteotomy was performed. 3.5 mm holes were predrilled for later reattachment. Aiming toward the medial corner of the tibial plafond at a 45° plane from the articular surface, the osteotomy cut was made. The fracture site was then clearly visualized and reduced using small K-wires to manipulate the fragments into an anatomic position. Two K-wires were then driven across the fracture site from the nonarticular talar neck to hold the reduction. The reduction was then checked on lateral, Canale, and Broden's views to assure that it was anatomic. The position of the K-wires was also checked on these views to assist with directing the final screws. Rigid fixation was then obtained by drilling, tapping, and placing two 4.0 mm cancellous screw through the nonarticular talar neck. Maximum compression was obtained by placing these screws perpendicular to the fracture plane. Their length and position were checked on fluoro to ensure that they had not breached surrounding joints. The wound was thoroughly irrigated with normal saline and closed with interrupted 4.0 nylon stitches in a vertical mattress fashion. The wound was dressed with non-stick gauze, 4 × 4's, and sterile soft roll. A posterior plaster splint was applied and wrapped with an Ace bandage.

The tourniquet was let down. The patient was awakened from anesthesia and sent to the recovery room in stable condition. Dr. _____ was present and scrubbed throughout the procedure.

Part VI

Shoulder and Arm

Chapter 67

Diagnostic Shoulder Arthroscopy

Said Saghieh, M.D.

COMMON INDICATIONS
- Internal derangement, shoulder

POSSIBLE COMPLICATIONS
- Hemorrhage
- Iatrogenic cartilage injury
- Fluid extravasation
- Neuropraxia
- Infection

ESSENTIAL STEPS
1. Careful preoperative assessment (history, physical examination, radiographs, US/MRI)
2. Portals
3. Glenohumeral examination
4. Subdeltoid bursae examination
5. Closure of portals

OPERATIVE NOTE
Preoperative Diagnosis: Internal derangement, shoulder
Procedure: Diagnostic shoulder arthroscopy
Postoperative Diagnosis:
Indications: ___ year-old male/female who has been complaining of R/L shoulder pain of several months duration.

S. Saghieh et al. (eds.), *Operative Dictations in Orthopedic Surgery*,
DOI 10.1007/978-1-4614-7479-1_67,
© Springer Science+Business Media New York 2013

Description of Operation: The patient and surgical site were identified and marked in the preholding area. The patient underwent anesthesia per the anesthesia team. The shoulder was examined under anesthesia. Then, the patient was repositioned in the lateral decubitus on a bean bag with all bony prominences padded. The torso was rolled posteriorly 25°, axillary roll placed, and the arm was placed into a foam traction sleeve and suspended in 30° of abduction, 15° of flexion. Ten pounds of weight were used for traction. IV antibiotics were administered.

The shoulder area was prepped and draped in the usual sterile fashion.

Bone landmarks and portal sites were drawn with a marking pen. The posterior portal site was injected with epinephrine and a superficial 6 mm incision was made. The arthroscopic cannula was introduced with blunt trocar through the posterior capsule and into the joint. The trocar was replaced by the scope. The camera, the source light, and the inflow tube were connected to the sheath. Fluid pressure was kept at 40 mmHg.

The anterior portal was then established in the rotator interval under direct visualization. Spinal needle was introduced from the outside, identified from inside before incision was made and anterior cannula introduced.

The biceps tendon was visualized. With the probe inserted anteriorly, its glenoid attachment was tested and proved to be _____. The anterosuperior labrum was evaluated and was found to be _____. The superior glenohumeral ligament and the middle glenohumeral were identified. Next the subscapularis was evaluated and found to be _____ Then the anteroinferior labrum was tested with the probe and found to be _____ The inferior glenohumeral ligament was _____.

The rotator cuff interval was assessed as well as the intraarticular side of the rotator cuff (findings).

Finally the posterior labrum was also examined.

The scope was redirected into the subacromial space. The lateral portal was established. A shaver was introduced and a bursectomy performed. The rotator cuff was again evaluated from above (findings).

The acromion was seen and the acromioclavicular joint localized (findings).

The anterior cannula and the scope were removed and portals closed with nylon 3-0.

Sterile dressings and an arm sling were applied.

No intraoperative complications.

Staff was present and scrubbed for entire procedure.

Chapter 68
Arthroscopic Acromioplasty

Said Saghieh, M.D.

COMMON INDICATIONS
- Impingement syndrome

POSSIBLE COMPLICATIONS
- Hemorrhage
- Iatrogenic cartilage injury
- Iatrogenic rotator cuff tear
- Fluid extravasation
- Neuropraxia
- Infection

ESSENTIAL STEPS
1. Careful preoperative assessment (history, physical examination, radiographs, US/MRI)
2. Portals
3. Glenohumeral examination
4. Subdeltoid bursae examination
5. Bursectomy
6. Acromioplasty
7. Closure of portals

OPERATIVE NOTE
Preoperative Diagnosis: Impingement syndrome, ---Shoulder.
Procedure: Arthroscopic acromioplasty
Postoperative Diagnosis: Same
Indications: ___ year-old male/female who has been complaining of shoulder pain secondary to an impingement syndrome of

S. Saghieh et al. (eds.), *Operative Dictations in Orthopedic Surgery*,
DOI 10.1007/978-1-4614-7479-1_68,
© Springer Science+Business Media New York 2013

several months duration. The patient failed conservative treatment including physical therapy and steroid injection.

Description of Operation: The patient and surgical site were identified and marked in the preoperative holding area. The patient underwent anesthesia per the anesthesia team.

The patient was positioned in the lateral decubitus position on a bean bag with all bony prominences padded. The torso was rolled posteriorly 25°, axillary roll placed, and the arm was placed into a foam traction sleeve and suspended in 60° of abduction, 15° of flexion. Ten pounds of weight were used for traction. IV antibiotics were administered.

The shoulder area was prepped and draped in the usual sterile fashion.

Bone landmarks and portal sites were drawn with a marking pen. The posterior portal site was injected with epinephrine and a superficial 6 mm incision was made. The arthroscopic cannula was introduced with blunt trocar through the posterior capsule and into the joint. The trocar was replaced by the scope. The camera, the source light, and the inflow tube were connected to the sheath. Fluid pressure was kept at 40 mmHg.

The glenohumeral joint was explored and no pathology was noticed. The scope was retrieved.

The arm was brought to 30° of abduction and the arthroscopic sheath was reintroduced with the blunt trocar into the subacromial space. The trocar was moved medio-laterally to break adhesions.

The scope was reintroduced. The acromion was identified. The lateral portal was established 3 cm distal to the acromion in line with the posterior aspect of the acromioclavicular joint. A shaver was introduced and a bursectomy performed. The rotator cuff was again evaluated from above. No tear was seen.

A coblator was introduced from the lateral portal and used to clean the soft tissue from the undersurface of the acromion.

A 5.5-mm acromionizer burr was then introduced through the lateral portal, and used to resect the lateral edge of the acromion just medial to the portal, starting at a depth of about 5 mm anterior and tapering posteriorly. The burr was kept lateral to the acromioclavicular joint.

After completing the acromioplasty, coblator was used again to achieve hemostasis.

The scope was removed and portals closed with nylon 3-0.

Sterile dressings and an arm sling were applied.

No intraoperative complications.

Staff was present and scrubbed for entire procedure.

Postop Regimen: The arm is placed in a sling, and Codman pendulum exercises are begun on the first day.

Patient is encouraged to remove the sling as early as possible and resume his/her daily living activities.

Active-assisted range-of-motion exercises and isometric strengthening exercises for the deltoid and rotator cuff are begun within the first week. Light resistance exercises using elastic tubing are started the second week. Most patients have a full range of motion by 3 weeks, and supervised progressive exercises against resistance are instituted and continued for 3 months.

Chapter 69
Arthroscopic Rotator Cuff Repair

Muhyeddine Al-Taki, M.D.

COMMON INDICATIONS
- Rotator cuff tear, shoulder

POSSIBLE COMPLICATIONS
- Hemorrhage
- Iatrogenic cartilage injury
- Fluid extravasation
- Neuropraxia
- Infection
- Failure of repair

ESSENTIAL STEPS
1. Careful preoperative assessment (history, physical examination, radiographs, US/MRI)
2. Portals
3. Glenohumeral examination
4. Identification and debridement of the tear
5. Identification of the footprint and anchor placement
6. Passage of the sutures through the rotator cuff
7. Lateral row anchors
8. Closure of portals

S. Saghieh et al. (eds.), *Operative Dictations in Orthopedic Surgery*,
DOI 10.1007/978-1-4614-7479-1_69,
© Springer Science+Business Media New York 2013

OPERATIVE NOTE

Preoperative Diagnosis: Rotator cuff tear, shoulder
Procedure: Arthroscopic rotator cuff repair
Postoperative Diagnosis: Same
Indications: ___ yo male/female who has been complaining of R/L shoulder pain and/or weakness of several months duration.

Description of Operation: The patient and surgical site were identified and marked in the preholding area. The patient underwent anesthesia per the anesthesia team. The shoulder was examined under anesthesia. Then, the patient was repositioned in the lateral decubitus position on a bean bag with all bony prominences padded. The torso was rolled posteriorly 25°, axillary roll placed, and the arm was placed into a foam traction sleeve and suspended in 30° of abduction, 15° of flexion. Ten pounds of weight were used for traction. IV antibiotics were administered.

The shoulder area was prepped and draped in the usual sterile fashion.

Bone landmarks and portal sites were drawn with a marking pen. The posterior portal site was noted and a superficial 6 mm incision was made. The arthroscopic cannula was introduced with blunt trocar through the posterior capsule and into the joint. The trocar was replaced by the scope. The camera, the source light, and the inflow tube were connected to the sheath. Fluid pressure was kept at 40 mmHg.

The anterior portal was then established in the rotator interval under direct visualization. Spinal needle was introduced from the outside, identified from inside before incision was made and anterior cannula introduced.

The biceps tendon was visualized. With the probe inserted anteriorly, its glenoid attachment was tested and proved to be intact.

The rotator cuff interval was assessed as well as the rotator cuff. There was a complete tear of the supraspinatus.

The scope was redirected into the subacromial space. The lateral portal was established. A shaver was introduced and a bursectomy performed. The rotator cuff was again evaluated from above. The tear in the rotator cuff was identified. The edges of the cuff tear were debrided with the shaver. Following that, the footprint of the rotator cuff was treated with the burr to get to bleeding bone. One/two anchors were introduced through a lateral portal and the sutures from the anchors passed through the rotator cuff using a suture passer. The sutures were tied and subsequently passed through one/two laterally placed anchors.

Finally, an acromioplasty was performed with a burr.

The anterior cannula and the scope were removed and portals closed with nylon 3-0.

Sterile dressings and an arm sling were applied. The patient was transferred to the recovery room in good condition.

No intraoperative complications.

Staff was present and scrubbed for entire procedure.

Chapter 70
Arthroscopic Bankart Repair

Brian R. Wolf, M.D., M.S.

COMMON INDICATIONS
- Recurrent anterior/anteroinferior glenohumeral dislocations, usually secondary to a traumatic initial anterior dislocation

POSSIBLE COMPLICATIONS
- Recurrent instability from repair failure
- Nerve or vessel damage
- Articular cartilage injury
- Persistent pain
- Infection

ESSENTIAL STEPS
1. Positioning of patient in lateral or beach-chair position dependent upon surgeon's preferred technique. Shoulder evaluation under anesthesia to assess instability.
2. Identification of bony landmarks and portal positions and distension of the shoulder joint.
3. Diagnostic shoulder arthroscopy and identification of Bankart lesion and capsule laxity.
4. Mobilization of torn anterior labrum.
5. Anterior glenoid neck debridement to bleeding surface.
6. Placement of suture anchors along anterior edge of glenoid.
7. Passage of sutures through anterior capsulolabral complex.
8. Tying of arthroscopic knots if needed.
9. Irrigate joint and close portals.
10. Sterile dressing.

S. Saghieh et al. (eds.), *Operative Dictations in Orthopedic Surgery*,
DOI 10.1007/978-1-4614-7479-1_70,
© Springer Science+Business Media New York 2013

OPERATIVE NOTE
Preoperative Diagnosis: Recurrent anterior shoulder instability
Procedure: Arthroscopic Bankart repair
Postoperative Diagnosis: Same
Indications: ___ yo male or female with history and physical examination consistent with traumatic anterior shoulder dislocation with recurrent anterior shoulder instability and pain.
Description of Operation: The patient was identified as the correct person in the preoperative holding area, the operative extremity was marked, and the patient was brought into the operative suite and placed supine on the operating table. He was induced into general endotracheal anesthesia without difficulty and the patient was then repositioned for his surgical procedure. The patient was placed up in the beach-chair position with all bony prominences well-padded distally. The head was secured in the headrest as well. The patient was given IV antibiotics prior to the beginning of the procedure. Exam under anesthesia demonstrated grade 2 anterior instability, grade 1 sulcus, grade 0 posterior translation, and full range of motion. The patient's left arm was then prepped and draped in a normal sterile fashion. A time out was performed with the entire surgical team.

The bony landmarks were palpated and marked on the skin. A standard posterior arthroscopy portal was created and the camera was inserted into the glenohumeral joint. Under needle localization a rotator interval portal was created just above the subscapularis tendon. A diagnostic arthroscopy was performed. The superior labrum and biceps were normal. There was detachment of the labrum and capsule from the anterior portion of the glenoid from approximately 7 to 10 o'clock consistent with a Bankart lesion. A moderate amount of laxity of the anterior capsule was seen adjacent to the Bankart lesion. The posterior labrum was normal. The articular surfaces were normal other than a small posterior humeral head Hill Sachs lesion. The rotator cuff was normal. There was minor anterior and inferior synovitis but no punctuate hemorrhage.

A high lateral rotator interval portal was then created 1 cm off the anterolateral corner of the acromion under spinal needle localization. A skin portal was created and a pointed switching rod was used to penetrate the lateral rotator interval just above the long head of the biceps and just anterior to the supraspinatus. A cannula was placed here and in the posterior portal. The camera was placed in the high lateral rotator interval cannula to better visualize the Bankart repair.

Next, an arthroscopic liberator was used to elevate the anterior labrum and capsule off the glenoid in the area of the tear. The labrum was mobilized until muscle fibers of the subscapularis were identified and the labrum easily reduced to its anatomic position. The arthroscopic shaver was used to lightly debride the anterior glenoid to a bleeding bony surface.

A 3 mm biocomposite suture anchor was then placed at the inferior aspect of the prepared glenoid at 7 o'clock using a drill and guide. The anchor was single-loaded with number 2 suture. A grasper was placed from the posterior portal and used to hold the detached labrum in an anatomic position. A lasso suture passer was used to penetrate the detached anterior capsulolabral complex just inferior to the anchor around the labrum and grasping approximately 5 mm of capsule. One of the sutures from the anchor was shuttled through the tissue. The sutures were tied using arthroscopic knots. This was repeated with suture anchors at the 8:30 and 10 o'clock positions. This completed the fixation of the labrum. The adequacy of the repair along the glenoid was checked and there was excellent reapproximation and tightening of the capsular and ligamentous structures along the glenoid. The final pictures were obtained.

The cannulas were removed as well as the scopes removed. The wounds were then closed with nylon sutures, and the sterile dressings were applied with Adaptive, 4×4's, and Tegaderms. The patient was awakened from anesthesia. A sling immobilizer was placed over his shoulder, which he will retain in for 3 weeks. The patient was taken out of the operative suite to the post-op recovery room in excellent condition without any evidence of immediate complications.

No immediate complications.

Staff was present and scrubbed for entire procedure.

Chapter 71
Open Bankart Repair

Youssef El Bitar, M.D.

COMMON INDICATIONS
- First shoulder dislocation in young patients with high-risk activities
- Recurrent shoulder instability or dislocation
- Shoulder pain with apprehension
- Identification of Bankart lesion on MRI

POSSIBLE COMPLICATIONS
- Nerve injury: axillary, musculocutaneous
- Inadequate placement of anchor sutures
- Subscapularis tendon rupture with rotator cuff insufficiency
- Avulsion of capsular repair
- Wound infection
- Shoulder stiffness
- Recurrent instability

ESSENTIAL STEPS
1. Positioning
2. Deltopectoral approach
3. Subscapularis incision
4. Capsulotomy
5. Anchor placement and obliteration of Bankart lesion
6. Closure

S. Saghieh et al. (eds.), *Operative Dictations in Orthopedic Surgery*,
DOI 10.1007/978-1-4614-7479-1_71,
© Springer Science+Business Media New York 2013

OPERATIVE NOTE

Preoperative Diagnosis: Bankart lesion, right/left shoulder
Procedure: Open repair of Bankart lesion, rt/lt shoulder
Postoperative Diagnosis: Same
Indications: This is a young female/male athletic patient with a recurrent anterior shoulder dislocation, R/L.
Description of Operation: The patient was identified in the preoperative holding area. The affected upper extremity was marked. The patient was brought to the operating room. He/she received general anesthesia. IV antibiotics were administered.

The patient was placed in the beach chair position. A sandbag was placed under the medial border of the scapula. The head was supported by soft head rests and the ears were protected. All the other bony prominences of the lower extremities and the left upper extremity were protected by soft cushions. The shoulder and the surrounding area were prepped and draped in the standard manner, with the upper extremity draped free.

The standard anterior (deltopectoral) approach to the shoulder was used. A 10 cm skin incision was performed over the deltopectoral groove, starting just proximal to the coracoid process and going distally. The incision was deepened through the subcutaneous tissues and fat until reaching the deltopectoral fascia. A self-retaining retractor was applied to the wound. The cephalic vein was identified lying in the deltopectoral groove. The fascia was incised parallel to the deltopectoral groove exposing the cephalic vein. The plane between the pectoralis major muscle medially and the deltoid muscle laterally was developed, with the cephalic vein retracted laterally with the deltoid muscle. The self-retaining retractor was repositioned more deeply into the wound spreading the pectoralis muscle medially and the deltoid muscle laterally. The underlying conjoint tendon and the subscapularis tendon were identified. Hemostasis was secured at this point of the procedure.

The upper extremity was externally rotated to expose most of the subscapularis tendon and the musculotendinous junction. The upper border of the tendon was identified as well as the lower border at the level of the leash of vessels running transversely. A blunt clamp was inserted from distal to proximal between the subscapularis tendon and the underlying shoulder capsule.

The subscapularis tendon was tagged with two parallel rows of no. 1 Vicryl stay sutures, taken into the tendon around 2 cm from its insertion on the lesser tuberosity of the humerus. The tendon was divided between the two rows of sutures. The underlying shoulder capsule was exposed. The capsule was also tagged with two parallel rows of no. 1 Vicryl stay sutures and was incised between the two rows of sutures. The capsular incision was more medial than the subscapularis incision.

The underlying glenohumeral joint was exposed. A humeral head retractor was inserted into the glenohumeral joint, retracting the humeral head laterally for better visualization of the joint. The detached anteroinferior part of the glenoid labrum (Bankart lesion) was identified. No other pathology was noted. The attachment area of the anterior labrum on the anterior glenoid rim was debrided using a rasp instrument to roughen the edge and allow better healing of the labrum. The labrum was tagged on its original insertion on the anterior glenoid rim using anchor sutures, with the knots done away from the joint cavity. Three suture anchors were placed in the anterior rim of the glenoid at approximately the 2-, 4-, and 6-o'clock positions in the right shoulder, and the 6-, 8-, and 10-o'clock positions in the left shoulder. The stability of the repair was checked and was found to be adequate. The humeral head retractor was removed.

The wound was irrigated. The self-retaining retractor was repositioned to the superficial layer of skin. The capsule was then sutured with imbrication of its medial and lateral portions using no. 1 Vicryl sutures. The subscapularis tendon was sutured using no. 1 Vicryl sutures. The deltopectoral fascia was sutured using no. 0 Vicryl sutures. The wound was irrigated again. The self-retaining retractor was removed. The rest of the wound was closed in layers using no. 2-0 Vicryl sutures for the subcutaneous tissues and no. 4-0 Monocryl subcuticular sutures for the skin. A dressing was applied. A sling and swathe was applied to the upper extremity.

The patient was extubated in the operating room and was transferred to the post anesthesia care unit in good condition.

Staff was present and scrubbed during the procedure.

Chapter 72

Weaver-Dunn Acromioclavicular Reconstruction

Rola H. Rashid, M.D.

COMMON INDICATIONS

- Symptomatic acromioclavicular joint separation requiring operative stabilization

POSSIBLE COMPLICATIONS

- Anesthesia
- Postoperative pain
- Infection

ESSENTIAL STEPS

1. Patient positioning
2. Prepping and draping
3. Incision
4. Exposure of distal clavicle, coracoid, and coracoacromial ligament
5. Release of coracoacromial ligament from acromion
6. Stabilize distal clavicle with coracoacromial ligament
7. Wound closure

OPERATIVE NOTE

Preoperative Diagnosis: Acromioclavicular separation
Procedure: Weaver Dunn acromioclavicular reconstruction
Postoperative Diagnosis: Same

S. Saghieh et al. (eds.), *Operative Dictations in Orthopedic Surgery*,
DOI 10.1007/978-1-4614-7479-1_72,
© Springer Science+Business Media New York 2013

Description of Operation: The patient and surgical site were identified in the preoperative holding area. After transport to the operating suite, antibiotic prophylaxis was administered intravenously. After adequate anesthesia was obtained, the patient was placed in a semi-sitting beach chair position. The head and neck were safely stabilized and all bony prominences were well padded and protected. The forequarter was prepped and draped in standard sterile fashion. A strap incision in Langer's skin line was made from the posterior aspect of the distal clavicle toward the coracoid, approximately 1 cm medial to the AC joint. Full-thickness subcutaneous flaps were developed. The distal 2 cm of the clavicle was exposed subperiosteally. The deltoid attachment to the anterior aspect of the clavicle in this region was detached, and this flap of deltoid was retracted laterally. The abundant scar tissue was removed. The coracoid was identified as was the coracoacromial ligament, both the anterior and posterior bands. With the arm abducted and deltoid retracted, the coracoacromial ligament attachment under the acromion was noted. This was divided sharply. Number 1 Ethibond sutures were placed on the acromial aspect of the detached CA ligament. Mersilene tape was then passed under the coracoid and looped around the distal clavicle to act as a stabilization device prior to transfer of this coracoacromial ligament.

With the clavicle manually depressed maximally, the Mersilene tape was then sutured tightly. The knot of the Mersilene tape was placed anterior so there would be no prominence over the superior aspect of the distal clavicle. Two small pilot holes were placed into the distal clavicle following excision of the distal 1.5 cm. Through these two holes number 1 Ethibond diagonal sutures of the coracoacromial ligament were passed on the superior aspect and sutured into place.

The wound was thoroughly irrigated. The deltoid was reattached to the clavicle through bone holes. The deltotrapezial fascia was imbricated, all using 0 Ethibond interrupted sutures. Another round of irrigation followed by subcutaneous re-approximation and 3-0 Monocryl skin closure with Steri-strips was done. The sponge and needle counts were reported correctly twice. The patient's left upper extremity was placed in a sling.

The patient was awakened from anesthesia and taken to the recovery room in stable fashion.

No immediate complications were noted.

The staff member was present and scrubbed for the entire procedure.

Chapter 73

Inferior Capsular Shift

Mark L. Hagy, M.D.

COMMON INDICATIONS
- Symptomatic multidirectional instability

POSSIBLE COMPLICATIONS
- Documented emotional or psychological disturbances
- Glenoid dysplasia or hypoplasia
- Noncompliance with preoperative therapy regimens
- Neurologic injury to axillary/suprascapular nerves

OPERATIVE NOTE
Preoperative Diagnosis: Multidirectional instability
Procedure: Inferior capsular shift shoulder
Postoperativc Diagnosis: Same
Description of Operation: The patient was identified and brought to the OR and placed supine on the OR table. One gram of Ancef was given preoperatively. General anesthetic was induced without difficulty. Patient was elevated to the beach chair position. Extremities were well padded. The head was placed with the headrest padded and stabilized. The upper extremity was prepped and draped in a sterile fashion.

Incision is made from the coracoid process distally following the entire anterior axillary line. Subcutaneous dissection is carried out and the deltopectoral interval is identified. The cephalic vein is identified and carefully protected. Branches as identified are ligated. The vein is freed and carried laterally. Blunt dissection of the deltopectoral interval is then further carried out down to the

S. Saghieh et al. (eds.), *Operative Dictations in Orthopedic Surgery,*
DOI 10.1007/978-1-4614-7479-1_73,
© Springer Science+Business Media New York 2013

level of the pectolaris major insertion. Just medial to the insertion the biceps tendon is found within the bicipital groove. The proximal 2-cm of the pectoralis insertion is released to assist in visualization. Retractors are carefully placed to move the deltoid laterally and the pectoralis major medially. At this juncture the clavipectoral fascia is identified. The fascia is then divided vertically just laterally to the short head of the biceps. This fascia is further released proximally to the level of the coracoacromial ligament. Care is taken at all times to know the location of and avoid dissection or excessive retraction on the musculocutaneous and axillary nerves. At this point fascia overlying the subscapularis is removed.

The upper and lower borders of the subscapularis are identified. Once the borders are identified the arm is externally rotated and the superior two-thirds of the tendon is excised 2 cm medial to its insertion on the lesser tuberosity. The subscapularis tendon is then carefully divided from the underlying capsule. At this point electrocautery is used to create a horizontal incision between the upper two-third and lower third of the tendon. This is carried out until the superior portion is a mobile component. At this point #1 ticron sutures are placed in the free subscapularis tendon, and set aside. A periosteal elevator is utilized to free any remaining tendon from the capsule to facilitated capsular repair. A retractor is now placed inferiorly to protect the axillary nerve.

The capsule is then incised in a vertical fashion midway between the glenoid and humeral attachments. T his is carried out from the rotator interval distal to approximately the 6 o'clock position. A #2 ticron stitch is placed in the inferomedial corner of the capsule. Additional sutures are placed along this capsular limb progressing superiorly to the rotator interval. Each stitch is placed in a horizontal suture fashion. At this junction, intra-articular visualization is maximized. No labral or Bankart lesions are appreciated.

The arm is then externally rotated 25–30°. Prior to capsular shift a large horizontal defect in the superior capsule at the level of the rotator interval is closed with #2 ticron in a horizontal mattress fashion. Once this interval is closed, the medial capsule is shifted laterally by passing the previously placed inferior suture on the medial capsule laterally and superiorly up to the lateral limb of the capsule. The remainder of the sutures in the medial capsule is passed in a similar fashion until the medial limb is completely positioned deep to the lateral limb. With the arm held in 25–30° of external rotation the sutures are then tied from inferior to superior. When suturing is complete, external rotation motion is verified. Attention is then turned to repair the lateral capsular limb medially. This is performed with #2 ticron in a horizontal mattress format. The wound is copiously irrigated with normal saline.

The subscapularis tendon is then repaired. The previously placed retention sutures are used to reattach the tendon to its lateral portion. Care is taken to avoid over tightening the tendon during repair. The horizontal division is then closed with interrupted #2 ticron suture.

The wound is again thoroughly irrigated. Subcutaneous closure is achieved with 2-0 vicryl and subcuticular skin closure is carried out with 3-0 monocryl. Steri-strips are applied and the wound is covered with sterile 4×4 gauze and tegaderm. The patient is placed in a shoulder immobilizer.

The patient is awakened from anesthesia and taken to recovery without any obvious complications.

Dr._____ was present and scrubbed throughout the entire procedure.

Chapter 74
Mini-Open Rotator Cuff Repair

Firas Kawtharani, M.D.

COMMON INDICATIONS
- Rotator cuff tear without major retraction

POSSIBLE COMPLICATIONS
- Inadequate repair
- Recurrent tear
- Stiffness
- Infection
- Ulna nerve paresis

ESSENTIAL STEPS
1. Patient position—beach chair
2. Shoulder diagnostic arthroscopy—assessment of the tear from the articular side
3. Assessment of the tear from the bursal side, acromioplasty
4. Incision, exposure of deltoid
5. Split deltoid, hemostasis
6. Mobilize the tear
7. Repair tear
8. Repair deltoid
9. Repair of subcutaneous tissue and skin

S. Saghieh et al. (eds.), *Operative Dictations in Orthopedic Surgery*,
DOI 10.1007/978-1-4614-7479-1_74,

OPERATIVE NOTE

Indication: this is a ----year-old lady who has been complaining of pain and weakness in her R/L shoulder for xxx months/years. MRI revealed a significant full thickness tear of her supraspinatus. After thorough discussion of the pros and cons, and the possible complications, the patient elected to have her rotator cuff fixed.

Preoperative Diagnosis: Rotator cuff tear, R/L

Procedure: Diagnostic shoulder arthroscopy. Arthroscopically assisted rotator cuff repair.

Postoperative Diagnosis: Same

Description of Operation: The patient was identified in the preoperative holding area where the involved extremity was marked. He/she was brought to the operating room and underwent endotracheal general anesthesia. IV antibiotics were given. The patient was placed in the beach chair position and all pressure points carefully padded. The shoulder was prepped and draped and all landmarks were carefully outlined with a marking pen.

Through a standard posterior portal, 2 cm distal and 2 cm medial to the postero-lateral corner of the acromion, the scope was introduced into the glenohumeral joint.

A diagnostic arthroscopy was then performed. The labrum was found to be intact with no bankart or SLAP lesion. The biceps tendon attachment was also disease-free. The subscapularis muscle was intact. There was a full thickness tear of the supraspinatus tendon.

The scope was then repositioned into the subacromial space with the use of a blunt trocar. The subdeltoid/subacromial bursa was found to be thick and inflamed.

A second working portal was then made through a separate stab incision 2 cm distal to the lateral border of the acromion along the clavicle axis. Again, the tear of the supraspinatus was identified.

A shaver was introduced through the lateral portal and a bursectomy was performed. Bleeding was controlled with a coblator (Mitek).

A 6.0-mm arthroscopic burr was used to perform an anterior acromioplasty to decompress the cuff.

At this point, it was decided to proceed with the open part of the procedure; a 4 cm skin incision was performed centered over the lateral portal incision and along a langer's line.

Subcutaneous tissue was dissected sharply down to the level of the fascia of the deltoid muscle. The raphe separating the anterior and middle deltoid muscles was incised and the deltoid fibers were split. Attention was made to avoid extension of the split beyond 4 cm from lateral acromion edge to prevent any axillary nerve injury.

The rotator cuff tendon was identified and the arm was rotated internally and externally to allow the rotator cuff tear to be positioned beneath the deltoid split. The cuff was mobilized proximally and pulled toward its initial insertion on the humeral head. The footprint was prepared with a rasp at the edge of the articular surface.

Three anchors (type) were drilled into the humeral head directly distal to the foot print. The sutures were tied down to pull the rotator cuff to its initial insertion on the greater tuberosity. The repair was checked and was judged to be excellent.

Once this had been performed the wound was copiously irrigated with normal saline.

The wound was then closed in three layers with #2 Tycron to close the deltoid split. Subcutaneous layer was then closed with 2-0 Vicryl in a buried running fashion. The skin was then sutured closed in a subcuticular running fashion with 4-0 Monocryl. The posterior arthroscopic portal sites were then closed with 4-0 Monocryl. The wounds were then dressed with sterile dressings with Steri-strips over the lateral incision as well as Xeroform, 4 × 4 gauze, and Tegaderm. The patient was awakened, transferred to the PACU after an arm sling had been applied to the operated extremity.

Chapter 75

Large Rotator Cuff Tear: Repair

Youssef El Bitar, M.D.

COMMON INDICATIONS

- Shoulder pain
- Decreased shoulder range of motion affecting quality of life

POSSIBLE COMPLICATIONS

- Infection
- Heterotopic ossification
- Shoulder stiffness
- Failure of the repair
- Deltoid muscle detachment with weakness
- Axillary nerve injury

ESSENTIAL STEPS

1. Positioning
2. Deltopectoral approach
3. Complete visualization and inspection of the rotator cuff
4. Anchor placement and re-approximation of the freshened rotator cuff edges
5. Closure

S. Saghieh et al. (eds.), *Operative Dictations in Orthopedic Surgery*,
DOI 10.1007/978-1-4614-7479-1_75,
© Springer Science+Business Media New York 2013

OPERATIVE NOTE

Preoperative Diagnosis: Rotator cuff tear, right shoulder
Procedure: Open repair of rotator cuff tear
Postoperative Diagnosis: Same
Indications: This is a middle-aged male patient, who is a construction worker, with right shoulder pain affecting his work ability and his activities of daily living. Conservative measures, including NSAIDs, analgesics, physical therapy, and bracing, failed to improve his quality of life.
Description of Operation: The patient received general anesthesia. The patient was placed in the beach chair position. A sandbag was placed under the medial border of the scapula. The head was supported by soft head rests and the ears were protected. All the other bony prominences of the lower extremities and the left upper extremity were protected by soft cushions. The right upper extremity, right aspect of the neck and chest areas were prepped and draped in the standard manner, with the upper extremity draped free.

The standard anterolateral approach to the shoulder was used. A 6 cm skin incision was performed over the anterolateral aspect of the shoulder, starting at the anterolateral corner of the acromion and going medially ending just lateral to the coracoid process. The incision was deepened through subcutaneous tissues and fat until reaching the deltoid fascia. A self-retaining retractor was applied to the wound. The fascia was incised perpendicular to the skin incision, parallel to the fibers of the deltoid muscle. The dissection was then carried through the deltoid muscle by splitting its fibers medially and laterally exposing the underlying subacromial bursa. The self-retaining retractor was repositioned more deeply into the wound, spreading the deltoid fibers medially and laterally. Part of the deltoid attachment to the acromion was elevated subperiosteally to expose the anterior aspect of the acromion for better visualization of the subacromial structures. The subacromial bursa was excised to expose the underlying coracoacromial ligament and rotator cuff. Hemostasis was achieved at this point.

The upper extremity was taken into a full range of motion to inspect the rotator cuff. The cuff was found to have a full thickness tear at the level of the supraspinatus tendon insertion on the greater tuberosity of the humerus. The edges of the tear were debrided to get healthy tissue for repair. The footprint of the tendon on the humeral head was debrided using a dental burr. Two anchor sutures were inserted into the humeral head at the level of the debrided footprint, the sutures were passed into the rotator cuff, and the cuff was pulled laterally and tagged down on its original insertion on the humeral head and the sutures were tied. Then two lateral anchor sutures were inserted into the humeral head, and the sutures were passed into the rotator cuff lateral to the previously inserted sutures, forming a double row repair of the rotator cuff. The sutures were tied. The repair was checked by taking the arm into full range of motion and was found to be adequate.

The wound was then irrigated. The self-retaining retractor was repositioned to the superficial layer of skin. The detached part of the deltoid from the acromion was sutured back in place using no. 1 Vicryl sutures. The deltoid fascia was sutured using no. 0 Vicryl sutures.

The wound was irrigated again. The self-retaining retractor was removed. The rest of the wound was closed in layers using no. 2-0 Vicryl sutures for the subcutaneous tissues and no. 4-0 Monocryl subcuticular sutures for the skin. A dressing was applied. An arm sling was applied to the upper extremity.

The patient was extubated in the operating room and was transferred to the post-anesthesia care unit in good condition.

Chapter 76

Total Shoulder Replacement

Muhyeddine Al-Taki, M.D.

COMMON INDICATIONS
- Inflammatory or degenerative arthritis of the shoulder joint

POSSIBLE COMPLICATIONS
- Infection
- Loosening
- Pain
- Instability
- Glenoid fracture
- Humeral fracture

ESSENTIAL STEPS
1. Careful preoperative clinical and radiographic assessment
2. Patient positioning in the beach-chair position
3. Anterior deltopectoral incision
4. Arthrotomy, release, and exposure of the proximal humerus and, later on, the glenoid
5. Bony cuts, measurements, and trial components
6. Implants fixation
7. Closure

S. Saghieh et al. (eds.), *Operative Dictations in Orthopedic Surgery*,
DOI 10.1007/978-1-4614-7479-1_76,
© Springer Science+Business Media New York 2013

OPERATIVE NOTE

Preoperative Diagnosis: Arthritis, shoulder
Procedure: Total shoulder replacement
Postoperative Diagnosis: Same
Indications: ___ yo male/female who has been complaining of R/L shoulder pain of several months duration resistant to conservative treatment.
Description of Operation: The patient and the surgical site were identified and marked in the preholding area. The patient underwent anesthesia per the anesthesia team.

The patient was placed in the beach-chair position. A small towel is inserted behind the scapula to elevate the shoulder with the affected arm completely free off the edge of the table. The upper extremity was prepped and draped in the usual manner.

A 15 cm longitudinal anterior incision extending from the coracoid process superiorly to the lateral edge of the biceps muscle inferiorly is performed and deepened between the deltoid muscle and the pectoralis major. The cephalic vein is identified and mobilized laterally. The conjoint tendon is identified and the deltopectoral fascia incised to expose the subscapularis tendon. The biceps tendon is identified, tenotomized, and tagged with a suture. The deltoid muscle insertion on the humerus is partially released superiorly if needed to improve the exposure. The rotator interval is identified and opened and the dissection continued inferiorly through the subscapularis tendon 1.5 cm medial to its insertion on the lesser tubercle. The tendon edge is held with three vicryl sutures. The joint capsule is opened and dissection continued over the humeral neck posteriorly taking care to protect the axillary nerve as it travels around the neck inferior to the capsule. The humeral head is externally rotated to improve its exposure, and to protect the rotator cuff tendons. The superior aspect of the head is noted and the canal finder of the humerus is inserted. The humeral head cutting jig is assembled and the humeral cut completed taking care to protect the rotator cuff tendons. The humeral canal is reamed to the appropriate size. The last reamer is left in the humerus to protect it from fracture.

Attention is directed to the glenoid. The head retractors are applied to expose the glenoid fully. The glenoid is prepared using the appropriate reamers. The glenoid is sized and the appropriate glenoid trial component is inserted. The appropriate trial humeral component is inserted and a trial reduction is done.

Trial components are removed and the definitive components are fixed. A hemovac in inserted.

After thorough irrigation, the wounds were closed in a routine layered manner.

Sterile dressing is applied.

No intraoperative complications.

Staff was present and scrubbed for entire procedure.

Chapter 77

Open Reduction and Internal Fixation Three-Part Proximal Humerus Fracture

Brian R. Wolf, M.D., M.S.

COMMON INDICATIONS
- Displaced three-part proximal humerus fracture (using Neer classification)

POSSIBLE COMPLICATIONS
- Nonunion
- Infection
- Axillary nerve injury
- Cephalic vein injury
- Brachial plexus or axillary artery injury
- Hardware failure

ESSENTIAL STEPS
1. Beach chair position
2. Anterior deltopectoral approach to shoulder
3. Mobilization and reduction of fracture fragments
4. Placement of internal fixation
5. Assessment of fixation and fracture stability
6. Wound closure and splinting

OPERATIVE NOTE
Preoperative Diagnosis: Displaced three-part proximal humerus fracture
Procedure: ORIF three-part proximal humerus fracture

S. Saghieh et al. (eds.), *Operative Dictations in Orthopedic Surgery*,
DOI 10.1007/978-1-4614-7479-1_77,
© Springer Science+Business Media New York 2013

Postoperative Diagnosis: Same

Indications: ____ yo male or female sustaining displaced three-part proximal humerus fracture

Description of Operation: Patient was brought to the operating room and positioned supine on the operating table with all bony prominences padded. General anesthesia was induced. A Foley catheter was placed under sterile technique. IV antibiotics were administered intravenously. She was then placed in a beach chair position with care taken to protect his or her nonoperative extremities. Fluoroscopy was positioned at the head of the table and views were checked to confirm the ability to visualize the proximal humerus. The left upper extremity was prepped and draped in the standard sterile fashion. A multidisciplinary time-out was performed.

The bony landmarks were marked on the skin and a formal deltopectoral approach was used. A 14 cm incision was made from the coracoid process to the deltoid insertion. The subcutaneous layer was dissected sharply, using a Colorado tip cautery, to the fascial layer. The saphenous vein was identified and dissected free through its entire course. No injury to the vein was sustained. The vein was retracted laterally with the deltoid as the deltopectoral interval was opened. Using blunt finger dissection, the undersurface of the deltoid was isolated from its origin on the acromion to the insertion on the humerus. The pectoralis major was retracted medially and the clavipectoral fascia was incised longitudinally, along the lateral border of the conjoined tendon. Again, blunt finger dissection between the coracobrachialis and subscapularis tendon allowed for identification and palpation of the axillary nerve and posterior circumflex humeral artery. The rotator interval proximal to the subscapularis was incised horizontally to allow visualization into the joint.

The distal dissection was performed using a cautery to identify the junction of the deltoid insertion and pectoralis major insertion. The biceps tendon was then palpated, starting distally and extending proximally, to identify our biceps groove and rotator cuff interval. The soft tissues on the medial side of the proximal humerus were grossly intact and dissection was avoided in this region, to protect the vascular supply to the humeral head. The greater tuberosity fracture fragment was palpated, and the fracture line was carefully identified, using a #15 blade to incise the overlying soft tissue and gentle Cobb elevation of the fracture margins.

The dissection was extended around the greater tuberosity fragment, on the medial side, just lateral to the biceps groove.

Again, the groove was not entered. The biceps tendon was then visualized through the rotator cuff interval and retracted medially. The greater tuberosity fragment was isolated and mobilized. The intra-articular surfaces were evaluated and there were no obvious injuries to the articular surface. The lesser tuberosity was in continuity with the humeral head.

The fractured greater tuberosity was reduced and provision fixation was performed with K-wires from lateral to medial. The head fragment next was reduced to the shaft with K-wires placed from the tuberosity into the shaft inferiorly. Fluoroscopy confirmed near-anatomic reduction. Next, an appropriate length proximal humerus locking plate was placed on the anterolateral side of the proximal humerus. The multiple proximal screw holes in the plate were then filled with a combination of 4.0 mm fully threaded cancellous screws and 4.5 mm locking screws using the guide system affixing the reduced tuberosities to the articular fragment. The shaft was secured to the head fragments by filling the distal screw holes with bicortical 3.5 mm screws in compression mode as needed. The shoulder was taken through a range of motion, including a forward flexion to 170°, without evidence of motion of the fracture site. Fluoroscopy confirmed appropriate reduction and hardware placement. Multiple views of the shoulder confirmed that no screws were prominent into the joint.

The joint was thoroughly irrigated through the rotator interval and the wound was copiously irrigated. The rotator interval was repaired and closed, with two 0-Vicryl sutures in simple fashion with the arm externally rotated to avoid overconstraint. The biceps tendon was visualized and protected with every throw of the suture through this interval. The subscapularis tendon was tethered with a #2 Ethibond to the supraspinatus tendon above the area of the tuberosity fracture.

The wound was again irrigated copiously with normal saline. A #2 permanent marking stitch was placed in the deltopectoral interval and cut long for future identification if needed. The saphenous vein was checked and was intact in its entirety at the time of closure. The subcutaneous layer was closed with 2-0 Vicryl in interrupted fashion, followed by a running Monocryl for the skin closure. Steri-strips, Xeroform, and 4×4s were applied, followed by a bulky sterile dressing.

The patient was awakened from anesthesia in stable condition, and transferred to recovery.

No immediate complications were noted.

Staff was present and scrubbed for entire procedure.

Chapter 78

Closed Reduction and Pinning of Two Part Proximal Humerus Fracture

Robert Frangie, M.D.

COMMON INDICATIONS
- Two parts displaced fracture of the proximal humerus

POSSIBLE COMPLICATIONS
- Nonunion
- Malunion
- Shoulder stiffness
- Loss of reduction
- Hardware failure
- Possible need to convert to open reduction
- Avascular necrosis of proximal humerus in anatomic neck fractures
- Neurovascular structure injury

ESSENTIAL STEPS
1. Closed reduction
2. Fluoroscopic confirmation of reduction
3. Pin placement under fluoro guidance

S. Saghieh et al. (eds.), *Operative Dictations in Orthopedic Surgery*,
DOI 10.1007/978-1-4614-7479-1_78,
© Springer Science+Business Media New York 2013

OPERATIVE NOTE

Preoperative Diagnosis: Two parts right/left proximal humerus fracture

Procedure: Closed reduction and percutaneous fixation of two parts right/left proximal humerus fracture

Postoperative Diagnosis: Same

Indication: ___-year-old male/female who fell down and sustained two parts right/left proximal humerus displaced fracture.

Description of Operation: The patient was identified in the presurgical area and the surgical site was marked. He/she was brought into the operating room and placed in a supine position. General endotracheal anesthesia was performed by the anesthesia team. IV antibiotics (name and dose) were administered. The patient was positioned in the beach chair position, and all pressure points were padded. The C-arm unit is positioned parallel to the patient from the head of the bed so that it does not interfere with movement of the arm. Closed reduction was performed under fluoroscopic guidance.

The shoulder and entire arm were then prepped and draped in a sterile fashion. Using C-arm the path of the Steinman pin (note size) was drawn and the skin entry site was incised.

A straight clamp was used to spread down to the humeral shaft. The pin was then introduced through the lateral cortex of the humerus shaft. It was driven up into the humeral head, as visualized under fluoroscopy in two planes.

A second similar pin was introduced parallel to the first one.

A third pin was directed downward from the greater tuberosity toward the medial cortex of the proximal shaft.

The pins were bent 90° at skin level and cut, then dressed with sterile gauze. The arm was placed in a sling. The patient was positioned supine and awakened from anesthesia. The patient was transported to the recovery room in satisfactory condition. There were no immediate complications associated with the procedure (or list complication and describe treatment or action taken, if any).

A staff was present and scrubbed for the procedure.

Chapter 79

Hemiarthroplasty of Shoulder

Ali Shamseddeen, M.D.

COMMON INDICATIONS

- Four part fractures of the humeral head where avascular necrosis is likely
- Head-splitting fracture with destruction of the articular surface
- Osteonecrosis of the humeral head without glenoid involvement
- More than 60 % of articular surface Hill-Sachs defect
- Osteoarthritis if glenoid cannot support a glenoid prosthesis
- Cuff tear arthropathy
- Metastatic tumor

POSSIBLE COMPLICATIONS

- Shoulder instability (anterior most common)
- Joint overstuffing
- Tuberosity nonunion
- Neurologic injury
- Infection
- Fracture
- Component loosening

ESSENTIAL STEPS

1. Beach chair positioning
2. Deltopectoral approach
3. Dislocation of the glenohumeral joint
4. Resection of humeral head
5. Reaming of the canal
6. Sizing of components

S. Saghieh et al. (eds.), *Operative Dictations in Orthopedic Surgery*,
DOI 10.1007/978-1-4614-7479-1_79,
© Springer Science+Business Media New York 2013

7. Placement of permanent components
8. Attachments of the tuberosities
9. Relocation of glenohumeral joint
10. Wound irrigation and closure

OPERATIVE NOTE

Preoperative Diagnosis: Four fragments shoulder fracture, R/L

Procedure: Shoulder hemiarthroplasty, R/L

Postoperative Diagnosis: Same

Indications: The patient is a ___-year-old male or female who sustained a four fragments displaced proximal humerus fracture, R/L. The patient was indicated for shoulder hemiarthroplasty after the risks of the procedure were clearly explained to the patient.

Description of Operation: The patient was identified in the preoperative holding area and brought to the operating room after marking the affected extremity. Under general anesthesia, brachial plexus block was carried for control of postoperative pain. The patient was then positioned in a beach chair position, the head was secured and all pressure points were appropriately padded. The upper extremity was prepped and draped in the usual sterile fashion.

A 15 cm longitudinal anterior incision extending from the coracoid process superiorly to the lateral edge of the biceps muscle inferiorly was performed and deepened between the deltoid muscle and the pectoralis major. The cephalic vein was identified and mobilized laterally. The conjoint tendon was identified and the deltopectoral fascia incised to expose the subscapularis tendon. The biceps tendon was identified, tenotomized, and tagged with a suture. The deltoid muscle insertion on the humerus was partially released to improve the exposure. The rotator interval was identified and opened and the dissection continued inferiorly through the subscapularis tendon 1.5 cm medial to its insertion on the lesser tubercle. The tendon edge is held with three vicryl sutures.

The joint capsule was found opened and the bone fragments were identified.

The head fragment was removed and the tuberosities were identified and tagged by heavy sutures. The proximal humerus was brought anteriorly and the humeral canal was then reamed till the appropriate size. The component sizing was then carefully performed and after placement of a temporary component and determining appropriate movement of the shoulder, a [name of component] was impacted into the proximal humerus and a size ___ modular humeral head was then carefully attached.

The component was put in 30° of retroversion, with preservation of the original humeral height by placing the component 3–5 mm above the level of the original tuberosities. The tuberosities fragments were then reattached to the prosthesis and the latter was relocated into the joint. The movement was noted to be normal in all directions with abduction up to about ___ degrees, at least 70° of internal rotation and 40° of external rotation in the abducted position of the arm were achieved. The anterior capsule was then carefully reapproximated with sutures going through the proximal humerus and then into the medial aspect of the capsule. The wound was then carefully irrigated with normal saline, and the subcutaneous tissue was closed with 2-0 Vicryl, and the wound was finally closed with 4-0 Monocryl after placement of a Hemovac. Dressings consisted of a layer of Xeroform and Kerlex and finally Tegaderm. A shoulder immobilizer was applied.

The patient was extubated and transferred to the recovery room with no complications.

A staff was present and scrubbed during the procedure.

Chapter 80

Antegrade Intramedullary Nailing: Humerus Shaft Fractures

Hamdi G. Sukkarieh, M.D.

COMMON INDICATIONS

- Displaced fractures of the humerus shaft
- Proximal fourth to the distal fourth
- Transverse or segmental
- Floating elbow injuries
- Fractures associated with thermal burns
- Fractures in the polytrauma patient
- A pathologic or impending pathological fracture may be the overall best indication for humeral nailing

POSSIBLE COMPLICATIONS

- Nonunion
- Infection
- Thermal necrosis with reaming
- Shoulder pain
- Loss of motion
- Subacromial impingement and rotator cuff irritation
- Iatrogenic fractures at the insertion site
- Iatrogenic comminution and distraction at the fracture site
- Risk to the radial nerve in the spiral groove from canal preparation and nail insertion
- Risk to the axillary nerve from proximal interlocking screws
- Risk to the radial musculocutaneous and median nerves, as well as brachial artery from distal interlocking

S. Saghieh et al. (eds.), *Operative Dictations in Orthopedic Surgery*,
DOI 10.1007/978-1-4614-7479-1_80,
© Springer Science+Business Media New York 2013

ESSENTIAL STEPS

1. Modified beach chair position on a radiolucent operating table
2. The base of the c-arm is positioned at the foot of the bed, parallel to the operating table
3. Starting point: just medial to the greater tuberosity and posterior to the bicipital tuberosity
4. Reduction of the fracture by a combination of adduction, neutral forearm rotation and traction
5. Guide wire down canal, checking AP and lateral alignment, take care to make sure wire is centered well in distal fragment
6. Open medullary canal with awl
7. Measure nail length and diameter
8. Reaming is performed in 0.5-mm increments until 1.5 mm of cortical chatter is achieved
9. A fracture gap should be avoided when nailing due to the potential of iatrogenic injury to the radial nerve
10. Proximally lock the nail with targeting device
11. Rotational alignment must be confirmed before static distal interlocking is performed
12. The fracture can be compressed after proximal interlocking by tapping the insertion bolt with the mallet
13. Distal interlocking screws inserted from an anterior-to-posterior direction are preferred because they avoid the radial nerve, which is more lateral

OPERATIVE NOTE

Preoperative Diagnosis: Humerus shaft fracture

Procedure: Antegrade intramedullary nailing, humerus shaft

Postoperative Diagnosis: Same

Indication: This is a ___year-old M/F who sustained a displaced humerus shaft fracture.

Description of Operation: The patient was identified and the site of surgery confirmed. Under general anesthesia, with the patient in the modified beach chair position on a radiolucent table, the affected upper extremity chest and neck were shaved, prepped, and draped in the usual sterile fashion. All bony prominences were padded. Prophylactic intravenous antibiotics were given. Fluoroscopy was brought in to confirm visualization of the entire humerus in the AP and lateral planes and a closed reduction was performed. The surface anatomy was palpated and outlined. The humeral head diameter was palpated from anterior to posterior to locate the midline. A 3-cm longitudinal incision was made from the edge of the acromion and carried distally. The deltoid muscle was split in line with its fibers. The subacromial bursa was cleared bluntly with finger dissection. An incision was made in line with the fibers of the supraspinatus tendon, and the tendon edges were retracted. A curved awl was used to initiate the starting point just medial to the greater tuberosity and posterior to the bicipital tuberosity. The awl was advanced into the intramedullary canal. Satisfactory position of the awl was confirmed fluoroscopically. A ball-tipped guide wire, visualized via fluoroscopy, was inserted and passed down the medullary canal. Reaming was performed in 0.5-mm increments until 1.5 mm of cortical chatter was achieved. The nail was securely attached to the alignment and driving guide. With the reduction held firmly, the guide wire was removed, and the nail carefully inserted by hand. The nail was driven below the cortical surface of the humeral head. Drill guides are placed through the alignment guide to mark the skin for small stab incisions used to insert the proximal interlocking screws. The soft tissues were gently spread down to bone using a hemostat to ensure a safe screw path. The drill sleeve and trocar were inserted through the guide and advanced to bone with gentle taps from a mallet. Interlocking screws of the appropriate length were inserted after drilling and measuring. A freehand technique was used to target the distal interlocking screws. Under fluoroscopy, a scalpel was placed over the skin to locate precisely the incision. An incision was made and a blunt hemostat was used to spread the brachialis muscle down to the bone. The drill bit was positioned perpendicular to the nail and the bone was drilled. The distal locking screws were placed after measurement. All wounds were irrigated thoroughly. A formal side-to-side rotator cuff repair is performed using nonabsorbable sutures. The deltoid raphe is also repaired. The deep fascia was approximated with 0-vicryl, the subcutaneous tissues with 2-0 vicryl, and the skin with staples. Dressings were applied. No complications were encountered and the patient was awakened and taken to recovery in stable condition.

Postoperative Management: The arm is placed in a sling or shoulder immobilizer at the end of surgery. After 2 days, gentle shoulder pendulum and elbow range-of-motion exercises are initiated.

Postoperative rehabilitation is tailored to the method of nailing, fracture stability, and overall patient health. Patients are seen at 2 weeks for suture removal, with subsequent follow-up at 4- to 6-week intervals.

Chapter 81
Biceps Tenodesis

Said Saghieh, M.D.

COMMON INDICATIONS
- Impending or acute rupture of the long head of the biceps

POSSIBLE COMPLICATIONS
- Persistent pain
- Failure of tenodesis (50 % failure in patient's diagnosed with bicipital tendonitis)
- Infection

ESSENTIAL STEPS
1. Beach chair positioning
2. Shoulder arthroscopy with debridement of the intraarticular portion long head of biceps
3. Identification of distal portion of biceps tendon
4. Incision just anterior and distal to acromion to expose intertubercular groove
5. Delivery of retracted tendon into proximal incision
6. Tenodesis of tendon to intertubercular groove with nonabsorbable sutures
7. Wound irrigation and closure
8. Placement of a sling

OPERATIVE NOTE
Preoperative Diagnosis: Impending or acute rupture of the long head of the biceps
Procedure: Shoulder arthroscopy, long head of biceps tenodesis
Postoperative Diagnosis: Same

S. Saghieh et al. (eds.), *Operative Dictations in Orthopedic Surgery*,
DOI 10.1007/978-1-4614-7479-1_81,
© Springer Science+Business Media New York 2013

Indications: __ year-old male or female with
   1. Acute rupture of proximal biceps with obvious deformity
      and distal migration of the biceps muscle. Pt has tender-
      ness anteriorly about the shoulder and weakness with
      supination.
   2. Pain and tenderness anteriorly about the shoulder. Speed's
      test (resisted elevation of the supinated arm with elbow
      extended) and Yeargerson's test (resisted supination with
      elbow flexed) were positive. Nonoperative treatment includ-
      ing physical therapy and NSAIDs were unsuccessful.

Description of Operation: The patient was placed supine on the
operative table. GETA performed by the anesthesia team. IV antibiotics were administered. The patient was positioned in the beach
chair position with head secured and all bony and soft tissue areas
well padded. The _____ upper extremity was prepped and draped
in the usual sterile fashion.

Shoulder arthroscopy was performed. Sixty cubic centimeter
of sterile NS was injected into the joint using a spinal needle. An
11 blade was used to incise skin in the standard posterior portal
(approximately 2 cm inferiorly and 1 cm lateral to posterior lateral corner of acromion). A blunt trochar was used to enter the
joint and the arthroscope was placed into the sleeve. An anterior
outflow portal was established using the variees needle. Shoulder
arthroscopy was performed. Using a moderately aggressive shaver
the proximal intraarticular stump of the long head of the biceps
was debrided. The shoulder was irrigated and the instruments
removed.

Next attention was turned to the distal stump of the biceps
tendon. A 3 cm incision was made over the deltobicipital groove
at the mid-arm to locate the distal portion of the tendon. The
tendon was identified and carefully freed with scissors and tagged
with nonabsorbable suture. A second 3–4 cm incision was made
just anterior and distal to the acromion to expose the intertu-
bercle groove. Using careful blunt dissection a tunnel was made
from the proximal to distal incision. A suture passer was placed
in the proximal incision and maneuvered into the distal incision.
The retracted tendon was delivered into the proximal incision. The
intertubercular groove was prepared using a burr to decorticate
the area lightly. Two suture anchors were placed in the middle of
the intertubercular groove. The tendon was secured using #2 nonabsorbable mattress sutures. The wound was irrigated copiously.
Wound was closed using 2-0 nondyed vicryl and 3-0 monocryl.
Steri-strips were placed and sterile dressings applied. The shoulder
was placed into a sling. Patient was extubated in the OR, moved to

the cart, and taken to the recovery room in satisfactory condition. Postoperative activity restrictions: sling 10–14 days, then advance to active shoulder ROM with avoidance of active biceps use for 4 weeks. Resistive exercise may begin after 10 weeks.

No intraoperative complications.

Staff was present for entire procedure.

Part VII
Elbow, Forearm, and Wrist

Chapter 82
Distal Humerus Open Reduction and Internal Fixation

Ali Shamseddeen, M.D.

DIAGNOSIS
Right supracondylar humerus fracture

Common Indications
- Intraarticular displaced fractures
- >1 cm displaced epicondylar fractures
- >20° of condyle/shaft angle loss in extraarticular fractures

POSSIBLE COMPLICATIONS
- Infection
- Malunion
- Nonunion
- Elbow stiffness
- Heterotopic ossification
- Posttraumatic arthritis

ESSENTIAL STEPS
1. Prone or lateral decubitus position
2. Radiolucent table
3. Posterior approach
4. Ulnar nerve exploration
5. Olecranon osteotomy
6. Fracture reduction and repair
7. Repair of olecranon osteotomy
8. Ulnar nerve transposition
9. Closure of wound

S. Saghieh et al. (eds.), *Operative Dictations in Orthopedic Surgery*,
DOI 10.1007/978-1-4614-7479-1_82,
© Springer Science+Business Media New York 2013

OPERATIVE NOTE

Preoperative Diagnosis: Right/left intraarticular supracondylar humerus fracture

Procedure: Open reduction internal fixation of the right/left supracondylar humerus fracture ulnar nerve transposition

Postoperative Diagnosis: Same

Indications: Comminuted displaced intraarticular supracondylar right humerus fracture.

Description of Operation: The patient was identified in the preoperative holding area and brought to the operating room. General endotracheal anesthesia was administered and IV antibiotics given.

The patient was put in lateral decubitus position with the upper arm supported by a padded post. The right/left elbow was then prepped and draped in the usual sterile fashion. A sterile tourniquet was applied to the proximal right arm. A longitudinal dorsal midline incision was made starting 15 cm proximal to the tip of the olecranon and extending over the proximal ulna for 4 cm.

The dissection was carried down to the triceps fascia and a medially based skin flap was elevated. The ulnar nerve was identified and dissected free of soft tissues and transposed medially. It was protected throughout this procedure using a vascular loop.

The triceps was then freed both medially and laterally. A chevron type olecranon osteotomy was performed using a power saw and an osteotome to complete the cut. The proximal olecranon and the triceps muscle were reflected proximally. This provided adequate exposure of the distal humerus and its intraarticular fracture pattern. The fracture was then copiously irrigated and the fragments were disimpacted and reduced to allow near anatomical approximation. There was marked comminution of the joint surface with fragments of the articular surface debrided. The medial and lateral condyles were fractured from the metaphyseal portion of the humerus with more lateral comminution such that anatomical fit of the lateral condyle could not be performed. The near anatomical alignment of the medial condyle, medial trochlear fragment, and lateral condyle and trochlear fragment was obtained and held with two single K-wires. The medial condyle was then anatomically reduced within the metaphyseal portion of the humerus and held with a 3.5 K-wire. The lateral condyle was also then held in a triangular fashion with a third K-wire to the distal humerus. A single 4.0 mm cancellous screw was driven across the medial condyle, medial trochlea, and lateral condylar fragments. This was not used in a lag fashion to prevent compression of the articular surface in regions of comminution. This trochlear reduction was obtained around the olecranoid semilunar notch for near anatomical approximation of the ulnohumeral articulation. Once this was completed attention was turned towards fixation of the distal humerus to the humeral metaphyseal region. Using 3.5 AO reconstruction plates appropriately bent, the medial condyle was secured to the proximal humerus. Screw fixation distally was of cancellous screws while proximal screw fixation was with bicortical screws. Finally the lateral column was secured with an appropriately contoured 3.5 recon plate applied posteriorly.

This provided a stable construct with flexion and extension of the elbow. The K-wires were removed and the wound was copiously irrigated. Flexion and extension of the olecranon, as well as passive forearm pronation and supination did not reveal any obvious blocks.

The olecranon osteotomy was then fixed with 2 K-wires and a wire loop applied as a tension band fixation.

All wounds were copiously irrigated. The ulnar nerve, which had been previously transposed medially, was secured medially and anteriorly using a fascia sling to prevent subluxation of the ulnar nerve posteriorly. All wounds were copiously irrigated. The subcutaneous tissues were closed with 2-0 Vicryl suture. 3-0 nylon in a horizontal mattress fashion was used to close the skin incision. Dry sterile dressings were applied as well as sterile soft-roll and a posterior splint was placed. The tourniquet was deflated.

The patient was extubated and transferred to the recovery room in stable condition.

An attending was scrubbed during the procedure.

Chapter 83
Elbow Arthroscopy

Hamdi G. Sukkarieh, M.D.

COMMON INDICATIONS

- Diagnosis and removal of loose bodies
- Evaluation and treatment of osteochondral injuries of the capitellum
- Excision of osteophytes from the coronoid and posterior olecranon
- Release of posttraumatic contractures of the elbow
- Synovectomy in inflammatory disorders
- Debridement of degenerative changes
- Evaluation of the ulnar collateral ligament and detection of valgus instability
- Evaluation of the painful elbow with uncertain intraarticular pathology

CONTRAINDICATIONS

- Elbow infection
- Severe bony or fibrous ankylosis or deformity
- Previous elbow surgeries that may affect neurovascular structure anatomy (ulnar nerve transposition)

POSSIBLE COMPLICATIONS

- Nerve or vessel damage
- Extravasation of fluid with acute capsular tear with risk of compartment syndrome
- Persistent pain
- Olecranon bursitis
- Infection

S. Saghieh et al. (eds.), *Operative Dictations in Orthopedic Surgery*,
DOI 10.1007/978-1-4614-7479-1_83,
© Springer Science+Business Media New York 2013

ESSENTIAL STEPS

1. Positioning of patient prone or supine-dependent upon surgeon's preferred technique.
   - Supine: hand placed into gauntlet or suspension unit in neutral position, 90° of abduction, and 90° of elbow flexion.
   - Prone: elevate the proximal arm and shoulder on a sandbag, shoulder 90° of abduction and 90° of elbow flexion.
2. Identification of bony landmarks and portal positions and distension of the elbow.
3. Establish the anterolateral portal first with skin incision, blunt dissection and trocar placement. Establish antero-medial portal under direct arthroscopic visualization.
4. Perform arthroscopy.
5. Irrigate joint and close portals.
6. Sterile dressing

OPERATIVE NOTE

Preoperative Diagnosis: One or more identified intraarticular elbow pathology as noted above

Procedure: Elbow arthroscopy

Postoperative Diagnosis: Same or list operative findings

Indications: ___ yo male or female with history and physical examination consistent with elbow intraarticular pathology refractory to nonoperative treatments.

Description of Operation: The patient was identified and the site of surgery confirmed. Under general anesthesia and IV antibiotics, and with the patient in the prone or supine position dependent upon surgeon's preferred technique; Supine: hand placed into gauntlet or suspension unit in neutral position, 90° of abduction, and 90° of elbow flexion. Prone: elevate the proximal arm and shoulder on a sandbag, shoulder 90° of abduction and 90° of elbow flexion. The operative arm was prepped and draped in the usual sterile fashion.

Bony landmarks about the elbow were identified with a marking pen and careful marking of the ulnar nerve. Inflate the tourniquet. 18 gauge needle inserted in the soft spot in the area of the direct lateral portal, and aimed directly at the center of the joint. The elbow was distended with 30-40 mL of fluid with a 50 mL syringe. Joint entry confirmed with visual distention of the joint and free backflow of fluid from the needle. Maximal distension of joint applied in order to anteriorly displace antecubital structures more anteriorly. A second spinal needle was then placed for the anterolateral portal and was used as a guide for cannula direction. Skin incision was made with an 11 blade. Straight hemostat used to spread the tissues to the level of the joint capsule. Joint was entered with a blunt trocar directed to the humerus palpating the medial epicondyle as the cannula was introduced and stabilizing the arm. The arthroscope was then introduced into the cannula without the fluid flowing to confirm intraarticular location. The anteromedial portal was next established under direct arthroscopic visualization. 18-gauge needle was placed 2 cm distal and 2 cm anterior to the medial epicondyle. This portal was established in the same fashion: skin incision, blunt dissection, and trocar placement.

Standard elbow arthroscopy was then performed. Additional portals direct lateral and straight posterior portal were established in the same fashion.

No immediate complications.

Staff was present and scrubbed for entire procedure.

Postoperative Management: A compressive dressing is wrapped around the elbow, and the patient is instructed to start using the elbow as tolerated. It is kept elevated when not in use for the first day to decrease swelling. If the procedure was performed for improving motion or for the treatment of arthritis, an indwelling catheter is inserted for brachial plexus block anesthetic if the neurologic examination is normal in the recovery room, and the patient is started on a full range of motion on a continuous passive motion (CPM) machine the same day. All circumferential dressings must be removed to avoid skin damage during CPM. Only an elastic sleeve is used to hold the absorbent dressing in place.

In general, debridement surgery of whatever type follows a similar postoperative course. Soft dressings are placed on the arm, and the patient is asked to begin immediate motion. In cases of stiffness, CPM can be utilized for the first 3–10 days.

Wrist curls without weights, elbow flexion, and extension exercises are started at 1 week, and resistive exercises begin at 2–3 weeks. If necessary, formal strengthening is initiated by 3–4 weeks postoperatively. The patient is allowed to resume normal activities as tolerated usually 3–12 weeks after surgery.

Chapter 84

Subcutaneous Ulnar Nerve Transposition

Said Saghieh, M.D.

COMMON INDICATIONS

- Cubital tunnel syndrome for more than 3 months despite postural care
- Periarticular fracture treated with open reduction and internal fixation
- Total elbow arthroplasty
- Valgus elbow with stretched ulna nerve

POSSIBLE COMPLICATIONS

- Ulna nerve injury
- Inadequate decompression
- Wound infection, dehiscence
- Elbow stiffness

ESSENTIAL STEPS

1. Skin incision.
2. Expose the cubital tunnel.
3. Isolate the ulnar nerve as it enters the cubital tunnel.
4. Follow the nerve proximally to the arcade of Struthers.
5. Excise the distal 8 cm of the intermuscular septum of the arm to prevent secondary impingement on the nerve after anterior transposition.
6. Decompress the nerve in the cubital tunnel.
7. Trace the nerve into the FCU muscle and divide the origin of the arch of the FCU.

S. Saghieh et al. (eds.), *Operative Dictations in Orthopedic Surgery*,
DOI 10.1007/978-1-4614-7479-1_84,
© Springer Science+Business Media New York 2013

8. Continue decompression of the nerve between the heads of the FCU, releasing Osborne's fascia, the fascia of the two heads of the FCU, and the pronator aponeurosis.
9. Divide the deep flexor pronator aponeurosis 8 cm distal to the medial epicondyle.
10. Mobilize the nerve from the cubital tunnel, preserving the small longitudinal vessels accompanying it.
11. Anterior transposition.
12. Closure.

OPERATIVE NOTE

Indication: This is ___ -year-old patient who has been complaining of numbness of the fourth, fifth fingers R/L over the past 6 months. EMG/NCT revealed the presence of severe compression of the ulna nerve at the cubital tunnel.

Preoperative Diagnosis: Cubital tunnel syndrome, R/L

Procedure: Decompression of the cubital tunnel.

Subcutaneous Anterior Ulnar Nerve Transposition, L/R

Postoperative Diagnosis: Same

Description of Operation: The patient was identified and the affected extremity was marked before transfer to the operating room. A regional block was administered by the anesthesiologist. IV antibiotics were given. A well-padded tourniquet was placed on the right/left proximal arm. The right/left upper extremity was then prepped and draped in the usual sterile fashion. The extremity was exsanguinated with an Esmarch and the tourniquet was inflated to 250 mmHg.

The arm was abducted in supination on a hand table.

A 12 cm curvilinear skin incision was made over the cubital tunnel, centered and slightly posterior to the medial epicondyle. The subcutaneous tissues were carefully dissected. The anterior skin flap was lifted to expose the common origin of the flexor muscles and the medial epicondyle. Care was taken to avoid damaging the medial antebrachial cutaneous nerve. The ulnar nerve was identified in its groove posterior to the medial epicondyle and freed of soft tissues. Using loupe magnification, the nerve was identified proximally to the cubital tunnel. A vessel loupe was placed around the nerve that was freed up to 8 cm proximal to the medial epicondyle. The medial intermuscular septum was excised and the arcade of Struthers was reached and released.

Distally, the nerve was freed by unroofing the cubital tunnel. It was followed between the two halves of the FCU where Osborne's band was incised. The superficial fascia was also released to a point 6 cm distal to medial epicondyle.

The nerve was exposed by blunt dissection of the muscle fibers taking care not to damage the motor branches. The flexor-pronator aponeurosis was tight and was released.

With the elbow flexed 90°, the nerve was transposed anteriorly to the medial epicondyle to lie directly on the fascia.

There was no kinking of the nerve in its transposed position.

A strip 2 × 2 cm of antebrachial fascia was raised at the medial epicondyle and reflected distally and laterally. It was sutured to the subcutaneous tissue anteriorly with 3-0 Vicryl to create a sling that prevents the posterior migration of the nerve.

The wound was irrigated. The subcutaneous tissues were approximated with 3-0 Vicryl. 3-0 Monocryl was used to close the skin in a subcuticular running fashion. The tourniquet was let down after a total of ___ minutes. Arm sling was applied.

The patient tolerated well the procedure and was transferred to the recovery room in stable conditions.

A staff was present and scrubbed during the entire procedure.

Chapter 85
Both Bone Forearm Fracture Open Reduction and Internal Fixation

Geoffrey F. Haft, M.D.

COMMON INDICATIONS
- Any displaced both bone forearm fracture in an adult
- Most open both bone forearm fractures
- Unreducable both bone forearm fracture in child
- Comminuted fracture

POSSIBLE COMPLICATIONS
- Infection
- Loss of forearm rotation
- Neurovascular injury
- Malunion
- Nonunion

ESSENTIAL STEPS
1. Volar approach to radial shaft
2. Longitudinal incision centered over fracture site
3. Identify interval between brachioradialis and flexor carpi radialis
4. Identify and protect radial artery and superficial radial nerve
5. Release muscle insertions from radius in subperiosteal manner
6. If fracture is proximal, care is taken to protect posterior interosseous nerve when releasing supinator
7. Fracture ends identified, cleaned, reduced anatomically
8. Fracture fixed using 3.5 LCDC plate
9. Ulna approached at subcutaneous border in interval between flexor carpi ulnaris and extensor carpi ulnaris

S. Saghieh et al. (eds.), *Operative Dictations in Orthopedic Surgery*,
DOI 10.1007/978-1-4614-7479-1_85,
© Springer Science+Business Media New York 2013

10. Fracture site identified and soft tissue cleared in subperiosteal manner
11. Fracture ends cleaned, reduced anatomically
12. Fracture fixed using 3.5 LCDC plate

OPERATIVE NOTE
Preoperative Diagnosis: Both bone forearm fracture
Procedure: ORIF both bone forearm fracture
Postoperative Diagnosis: Same
Indications: __yo patient with one of the indications above.
Description of Operation: The patient was identified in the preoperative holding area and the extremity was marked. The patient was taken to the operating room and placed supine on the operating table. He/she was given 1 g of Ancef IV. After adequate regional/general anesthesia was obtained, the arm was wrapped with an adequate amount of soft-roll and a tourniquet was placed. The arm was then prepped and draped in the standard sterile surgical fashion. The arm was exsanguinated with an Esmarch bandage and the tourniquet was raised to 100 mmHg greater than systolic pressure.

A volar approach to the radius was used. A 10 cm longitudinal skin incision, centered on the fracture site, was made along a virtual line extending from the anterior flexor crease of the elbow just lateral to the biceps tendon and extending distally to the styloid process of the radius. The incision was deepened through the subcutaneous tissue. The fascia of the forearm was incised in line with the incision. The medial border of the brachioradialis was identified and the interval between it and the flexor carpi radialis was incised. Proximally, the interval between brachioradialis and pronator teres was entered. The superficial radial nerve on the underside of the brachioradialis was identified and retracted laterally with the brachioradialis muscle.

The pronator teres and flexor digitorum superficialis were released from their radius insertions in a subperiosteal manner to visualize the fracture.

The ends of bone at the fracture site were stripped of soft tissue in either direction to allow for anatomic reduction. The wound was irrigated to clearly identify both bone ends. The fracture was reduced and held in place with a pointed tenaculum. A seven hole 3.5 LCDCP plate was then slightly bent to accommodate the curve of the radius. The plate was fixed into the volar side of the radius using standard AO compression technique. Three bicortical screws filled the three holes on either end of the fracture site.

The wound was then thoroughly irrigated with normal saline and closed in layers. The subcutaneous layer was closed with 2.0-Vicryl sutures in an interrupted, buried fashion. The skin was closed with staples.

Attention was then turned to the fractured ulna. An 8 cm linear longitudinal incision was made directly over the subcutaneous border of the ulna, centered over the fracture site. This was carried sharply to bone in the interval between the flexor carpi ulnaris and extensor carpi ulnaris. The periosteum of the ulna was incised longitudinally. The dissection was then carried subperiosteally around the volar surface of the ulna to uncover the fracture site. Care was taken to keep the dissection in a subperiosteal plane in order to protect the ulnar nerve. The ends of bone at the fracture site were stripped of soft tissue and callus 1–2 mm in either direction to allow for clear visualization of an anatomic reduction. The wound was irrigated to clearly identify both bone ends. The fracture was reduced and held in place with a pointed tenaculum. A seven hole 3.5 LCDC plate was then selected and fixed onto the ulna using standard AO compression technique. Three bicortical screws filled the three holes on either end of the fracture site. The wound was then thoroughly irrigated with normal saline and closed in layers. The subcutaneous layer was closed with 2.0-Vicryl sutures in an interrupted, buried fashion. The skin was closed with staples.

Both wounds were dressed with a nonadhesive dressing, 4 × 4 gauze, and sterile soft roll. A volar plaster splint was placed and wrapped with an Ace bandage.

The tourniquet was let down. The patient was awakened from anesthesia and sent to the recovery room in stable condition. Dr. _____ was present and scrubbed throughout the procedure.

Chapter 86

Distal Radius External Fixation and Percutaneous Pinning

Geoffrey F. Haft, M.D.

COMMON INDICATIONS
- Comminuted distal radius fracture
- Shortened distal radius fracture
- Gapped intraarticular distal radius fracture
- Stepped intraarticular distal radius fracture
- Some open distal radius fractures

POSSIBLE COMPLICATIONS
- Pin site infection
- Posttraumatic arthritis
- Superficial radial nerve injury
- Radial artery injury
- Other neurovascular injury
- Malunion
- Nonunion

ESSENTIAL STEPS
1. Incision at proximal, radial aspect of index metacarpal
2. Distal pins placed
3. Use fixator to judge position of proximal pins
4. Incision on dorsoradial aspect of radius
5. Protect superficial radial nerve
6. Place proximal pins
7. Attach fixator
8. Closed reduction to restore length, volar tilt
9. Tighten fixator joints

S. Saghieh et al. (eds.), *Operative Dictations in Orthopedic Surgery*,
DOI 10.1007/978-1-4614-7479-1_86,
© Springer Science+Business Media New York 2013

10. Use K-wires as necessary to joystick intraarticular fragments into acceptably reduce position
11. Place appropriate number of 0.062 in K-wires to secure fixation of reduced fragments
12. Bend and cut wires; ensure that skin is relaxed around wires

OPERATIVE NOTE

Preoperative Diagnosis: Comminuted, shortened distal radius fracture

Procedure: Distal radius external fixation and percutaneous pinning

Postoperative Diagnosis: Same

Indications: __yo patient with distal radius fracture

Description of Operation: Pt was taken to the operating room and placed supine on the operating table. She was given 1 g of Ancef IV. After adequate regional/general anesthesia was obtained, the arm was wrapped with an adequate amount of soft-roll and a tourniquet was placed. The arm was then prepped and draped in the standard sterile surgical fashion. The tourniquet was not used during the case.

First, a commercially available external fixation device was placed. A longitudinal incision was made over the proximal 1 cm of the radial aspect of the index metacarpal. The dissection was carried down bluntly to the anterolateral bone surface lying between the more dorsal extensor tendon and the more radial first dorsal interosseous muscle. Next, using a drill guide, a 2 mm drill was used to penetrate the proximal cortex of the metacarpal at its metaphyseal flare. The drilling was continued across the index metacarpal and into the base of the long finger metacarpal. A self tapping 3 mm half pin was then placed in the drill hole and its position checked with fluoro. The appropriate guide was then used to drill and place the second distal pin into the index metacarpal shaft. Next the external fixator was placed loosely over the distal pins to approximate the level of the proximal incison. About 10 cm proximal to the distal wrist crease, a 3 cm longitudinal incision was made along the mid-radial aspect of the radius. Dissection was carried bluntly through the subcutaneous tissue down to bone in order to protect the superficial radial nerve. The wrist extensor tendons were retracted dorsally and the brachioradialis volarly. Using the appropriate guide, two 2 mm bicortical drill holes were made and two 3 mm half pins were placed. The position of all pins were checked fluoroscopically. The skin incisions were then thoroughly irrigated and closed loosely around the pins with

4.0 nylon stitches. The external fixator was then applied tightly to the pins with the joints of the fixator left loose. A closed reduction was then performed by pulling traction on the index, thumb, and long fingers while placing volarly directed pressure on the distal segment of the fracture. With the traction maintained, the joints of the fixator were tightened and the reduction was checked with fluoroscopy. The radius was held out to length and the volar angulation of the distal segment was restored.

Attention was then turned to percutaneous pinning of the fracture fragments. This fracture had (number) of intraarticular fragments. There was initially a 2 mm stepoff at the articular surface between two of the fragments. This was reduced by placing a single 0.062 in. K-wire into the more radial fragment from a dorsal starting point and joysticking it into an anatomic position. The fracture fragments were then secured into place with two 0.062 in. K-wires. The first wire was fired from the radial styloid parallel to the joint surface, through subchondral bone, into the ulna. This wire skewered the large intraarticular fragments. The second wire was fired from the radial styloid in a distal to proximal, slightly dorsal to volar orientation across the transverse fracture site and through the ulnar cortex of the radius. The reduction and the placement of the wires was checked on orthogonal fluoroscopic views and felt to be satisfactory. The wires were bent and cut near the skin surface, and care was taken to ensure the skin was relaxed around the wires. The wires and pins were all wrapped with petroleum impregnated gauze. The pins were wrapped with dry gauze and the entire fixator was wrapped with an ace bandage.

The patient was awakened from anesthesia and sent to the recovery room in stable condition. Dr. _____ was present and scrubbed throughout the procedure.

Chapter 87

Open Reduction and Internal Fixation Distal Radius, Volar Approach

Ali Shamseddeen, M.D.

COMMON INDICATIONS
- When closed reduction fails to achieve adequate alignment
- Fracture is unstable

POSSIBLE COMPLICATIONS
- Infection
- Tendon rupture
- Regional sympathetic dystrophy
- Median nerve injury
- Malunion
- Nonunion

ESSENTIAL STEPS
1. Careful preoperative assessment
2. Volar approach
3. Reduction
4. 2.5/3.5 mm locking compression plate fixation
5. C-Arm verification

OPERATIVE NOTE
Preoperative Diagnosis: Distal radial fracture
Procedure: ORIF distal radius
Postoperative Diagnosis: Same
Description of Operation: The patient and surgical site were identified and marked. The patient underwent anesthesia per the

S. Saghieh et al. (eds.), *Operative Dictations in Orthopedic Surgery*,
DOI 10.1007/978-1-4614-7479-1_87,
© Springer Science+Business Media New York 2013

anesthesia team. The patient was positioned supine on the operative table with all bony prominences padded. A tourniquet was place on the arm over soft-roll. IV antibiotics were administered.

The upper extremity was prepped and draped as usual. The tourniquet was inflated to 250 mmHg.

A 7 cm straight incision was made over the volar aspect of the radius. It started at the joint line, on the lateral border of the flexor carpi radialis tendon. It was deepened through the subcutaneous tissue. The fascia of the FCR was incised and the tendon retracted medially. The radial artery was identified and retracted laterally.

The pronator quadratus was dissected off the lateral edge of the radius and retracted medially to visualize the fracture.

Reduction was achieved with manual traction and the use of small periosteal elevator. It was temporary maintained with 1.6 K wires.

The 2.5/3.5 mm LCP plate was applied. The first screw was a compression screw in the oblong hole to assure plate contact and adequate positioning of the plate.

Then the distal locking screws were inserted. Finally, two locking screws were added on the proximal side.

Final fluoroscopic verification showed adequate alignment.

Irrigation was done. Tourniquet deflated and hemostasis achieved.

Wound was closed in two layers: the subcutaneous tissue with vicryl 3.0 and skin with staples.

Dressing and a volar splint were applied.

No intraoperative complications.

Staff was present and scrubbed for entire procedure.

Post-op regimen: Volar splint is applied for 10 days then aggressive physical therapy.

Chapter 88
Wrist Fusion

Ali Shamseddeen, M.D.

COMMON INDICATIONS
- Posttraumatic arthritis with painful destruction of the joint
- Irreparable distal radial intraarticular fractures
- Joint destruction caused by infection or tumor resection, Kienböck disease, rheumatoid arthritis
- Stabilization of a paralytic wrist and hand
- Correction or wrist flexion deformity in patients with spastic hemiplegia
- Failed wrist arthroplasty

POSSIBLE COMPLICATIONS
- Painful hardware
- Nonunion
- Infection
- Tendon rupture
- Regional sympathetic dystrophy

ESSENTIAL STEPS
1. Careful preoperative assessment
2. The AO technique followed here uses the titanium dynamic compression plate
3. Above elbow cast till the distal fingers post-op is applied, elbow at right angle and forearm in neutral position, wrist in 10-year-old 15° of dorsiflexion

S. Saghieh et al. (eds.), *Operative Dictations in Orthopedic Surgery*,
DOI 10.1007/978-1-4614-7479-1_88,
© Springer Science+Business Media New York 2013

OPERATIVE NOTE

Preoperative Diagnosis: Wrist painful arthritis

Procedure: Wrist arthrodesis

Postoperative Diagnosis: Same

Description of Operation: The patient and surgical site were identified and marked. The patient underwent anesthesia per the anesthesia team. The patient was positioned supine on the operative table with all bony prominences padded. A tourniquet was place on the arm over soft-roll. IV antibiotics were administered. The upper extremity was scrubbed and draped in the usual fashion. A curvilinear incision was made over the wrist starting 2 cm proximal to the distal radioulnar joint and extending to the midshaft of the third metacarpal. The subcutaneous fat was incised to expose the extensor retinaculum. Incision of the extensor retinaculum was then carried, the plane between the extensor pollicis longus which was retracted radially, and the extensor digitorium communis which was retracted to the ulnar side was identified. The deep capsule of the radiocarpal joint and the carpometacarpal joints was then incised longitudinally. Dissection was continued below the capsule (the dorsal radiocarpal ligament) toward the radial and ulnar sides of the radius to expose the entire distal end of the radius and carpal bones. The tendons of the extensor carpi radialis longus and brevis were retracted radially to fully expose the Lister's tubercle which was removed using an osteotome. The articular cartilage was removed from both sides of the joint using small osteotomes, rongeur, and curettes.

The gaps were filled with bone graft. The precontoured 3.5 mm LCDCP plate was applied from the distal radius to the third metcarpal shaft maintaining the wrist in 30° of dorsiflexion.

__Screws were inserted in the third metacarpal and __ screws in the distal radius.

Irrigation was done, tourniquet deflated, and hemostasis achieved.

The wound was closed in anatomical layers. Small Hemovac drain applied.

Post-op regimen: Application of a long arm above elbow cast.

No intraoperative complications.

Staff was present and scrubbed for entire procedure.

Chapter 89

Wrist Arthroscopy

Abdel Majid Sheikh Taha, M.D.

COMMON INDICATIONS

- Synovial biopsy and synovectomy
- Chondroplasty and loose body removal
- Staging and debridement of avascular necrosis
- Ganglion resection: volar and dorsal
- Release of wrist contracture
- Treatment of interosseous ligament injuries: SLIL and LTIL
- Dorsal radiocarpal ligament repair
- Evaluation and treatment of carpal instability: scapholunate, lunotriquetral, midcarpal
- Triangular fibrocartilage tears: repair vs. debridement
- Arthroscopic wafer resection
- Arthroscopic bone resection: hamate pole resection, radial styloidectomy, distal scaphoid resection, proximal row carpectomy
- Reduction and internal fixation of distal radius fractures
- Arthroscopy-assisted fixation of scaphoid fractures
- Arthroscopic shrinkage of the trapeziometacarpal joint
- Arthroscopic hemiresection of the trapeziometacarpal joint with or without interposition substance
- Arthroscopic scaphotrapezial debridement or resection

POSSIBLE COMPLICATIONS

- Infection
- Nerve injury
- Edema

S. Saghieh et al. (eds.), *Operative Dictations in Orthopedic Surgery*,
DOI 10.1007/978-1-4614-7479-1_89,
© Springer Science+Business Media New York 2013

- Bleeding
- Scarring
- Tendon tearing

ESSENTIAL STEPS
1. Extremity positioned in abduction and traction applied through fingertraps
2. The joint is entered through a portal between the EPL and the EDC
3. The second portal is placed 1 cm ulnar and slightly proximal to the first portal
4. Scopes are retrieved
5. Skin closure

OPERATIVE NOTE
Preoperative Diagnosis: Wrist pain

Procedure: Wrist arthroscopy

Postoperative Diagnosis: Mention pathology noted intra-operatively

Description of Operation: Under regional anesthesia, the patient is positioned supine on the operating table. The arm is abducted and the fingers are suspended from 5 to 10 lb of fingertrap traction. The forearm and wrist are prepped and draped in the usual manner. Under tourniquet control, a 22-gauge needle is inserted in the space between the EPL and the EDC just distal to Lister's tubercle at 10° of proximal inclination. Then, 5 mL of normal saline is injected into the space. A superficial skin is done. The subcutaneous tissues are dissected bluntly using tenotomy scissors. The posterior capsule is pierced. Trocar and cannula are inserted. The scope is inserted. The RSL, RSC, SLIL, and LRL are visualized (Intra-operative findings). Then, a 22-gauge needle is inserted 1 cm ulnar and slightly proximal to the previous portal. A superficial skin incision and blunt dissection are done. The posterior capsule is entered. The ulnar half of the lunate, the TFCC and the ulnocarpal ligaments are visualized (intra-operative findings). Then, the trocars and cannulas are retrieved. The wounds are closed using 4.0 Nylon sutures. A sterile dressing is applied. Tourniquet is deflated. The patient tolerated the procedure well and left the operating theatre in good condition.

Staff was present and scrubbed during the procedure.

Chapter 90

Percutaneous Scaphoid Fixation

Firas Kawtharani, M.D.

COMMON INDICATIONS
- Nondisplaced transverse fractures of the waist of the scaphoid

CONTRAINDICATIONS
- Displaced fractures
- Distal or proximal pole fractures
- Oblique fractures

POSSIBLE COMPLICATIONS
- Failure of fixation
- Secondary displacement
- Nonunion

ESSENTIAL STEPS
1. Dorsiflex the wrist using rolled towels underneath it
2. Guidewire placement proximally through the volar scaphoid tuberosity
3. Screw measurement done through a second wire
4. Small incision around guidewire made
5. Drilling over the wire
6. Placement of the cannulated screw over the guidewire spanning the fracture
7. Proper placement and maneuvering done using the image intensifier
8. Wound closure and thumb spica splint applied

S. Saghieh et al. (eds.), *Operative Dictations in Orthopedic Surgery*,
DOI 10.1007/978-1-4614-7479-1_90,
© Springer Science+Business Media New York 2013

OPERATIVE NOTE

Preoperative Diagnosis: Nondisplaced scaphoid waist fracture, R/L

Procedure: Percutaneous fixation of scaphoid fracture

Postoperative Diagnosis: Same

Description of Operation: The patient was identified in the preoperative holding area. The affected wrist was marked. The patient was taken to the operating room and placed in the supine position with the arm abducted on a radiolucent arm table. Regional anesthesia was induced. Prepping and draping of the injured upper extremity was done.

Two rolled towels were used under the supinated wrist to allow for adequate dorsiflexion. Under fluoroscopy control, and with the wrist hyperextended, the guidewire for the cannulated screw system was placed through the volar scaphoid tuberosity, directed along the proximal aspect, dorsally, and ulnarly slightly diagonal to the longitudinal axis of the scaphoid and across the fracture site.

Next, a second guidewire was placed parallel to the first guidewire for antirotation control but far enough so it does not interfere with the drill or screw.

Screw length was measured with the use of a second guide pin.

A 3 mm incision is made around the guidewire followed by blunt dissection. Drilling and tapering is performed along the guidewire, up to the measured length. A cannulated screw slightly shorter than the measured length is inserted. Fluroscopy is used during this step to secure a good reduction and screw position. The fracture spanning and antirotation guidewires were removed.

The wound was closed with a 4.0 nylon suture. A well-padded, short arm thumb spica splint was applied. The patient was transferred to the recovery room in a stable condition.

Staff was present and scrubbed for the whole procedure.

Chapter 91

Treatment of Scaphoid Nonunion

Abdel Majid Sheikh Taha, M.D.

COMMON INDICATIONS

- Nonunion or delayed union of scaphoid fractures involving the waist and distal pole of the scaphoid
- No radiographic evidence of wrist arthritis or instability

POSSIBLE COMPLICATIONS

- Infection
- Scar
- Neurovascular damage
- Wrist stiffness
- Persistence of nonunion
- Wrist instability
- Wrist arthritis

ESSENTIAL STEPS

1. Volar wrist 5 cm longitudinal incision over radial aspect
2. Identifying and sparing neurovascular bundle
3. Arthrotomy and identification of nonunion
4. Harvesting of iliac crest bone graft
5. Debridement of nonunion
6. Bone grafting and reduction
7. Fixation of nonunion
8. Repair of capsuloligamentous structures
9. Skin closure

OPERATIVE NOTE

Preoperative Diagnosis: Nonunion of scaphoid fracture, R/L
Procedure: Repair nonunion of scaphoid fracture, R/L
Postoperative Diagnosis: Same

S. Saghieh et al. (eds.), *Operative Dictations in Orthopedic Surgery*,
DOI 10.1007/978-1-4614-7479-1_91,

Indications: The patient is an X-year-old m/w who had a fracture of the waist of the R/L scaphoid treated with cast for 4 months without evidence of healing.

Description of Operation: The patient was identified in the preoperative holding area. The affected extremity was marked. The patient was brought to the operating room and placed supine on the operating table with a bump under his/her l/r flank. A tourniquet was applied on the R/L upper arm.

After adequate anesthesia was obtained, the R/L upper extremity and the R/L flank were sterilely prepped and draped. The limb was exsanguinated with an Esmarch bandage and tourniquet inflated to 250 mmHg.

A longitudinal skin incision was made over the palmar surface of the wrist, beginning 4 cm proximal to the wrist flexion crease over the flexor carpi radialis and curved radially toward the scaphotrapezial and trapeziometacarpal joints. The terminal branches of the palmar cutaneous branch of the median nerve and the superficial radial nerves were identified and spared. The sheath of the flexor carpi radialis was opened. The tendon was retracted radially and the deep surface of its sheath was opened. The palmar aspect of the joint was identified. The wrist was extended in ulnar deviation and the capsule was opened along the longitudinal axis of the scaphoid bone, obliquely extending the incision toward the scaphotrapezial joint. The long radiolunate and radioscaphocapitate ligaments were incised, preserving each leaf of these capsuloligamentous structures for later repair. The nonunion was identified and debrided without damage to the cortical shell.

A 2 cm transverse incision was made over the R/L iliac crest. It was deepened through the subcutaneous tissue. The fascia was incised and the abdominal muscles reflected from their attachment. The periosteum was opened. The crest was identified. With an osteotome and curettes, corticocancellous bone graft was harvested.

The iliac crest wound was irrigated and closed in anatomical layers: the fascia with 0 vicryl, the subcutaneous with vicryl 2.0, and the skin with monocryl 4.0 in subcuticular fashion.

Reduction of the nonunion was performed. The harvested bone graft was contoured into a trapezoidal shape and inserted into the cavity to restore the shape of the scaphoid. The reduction was fixed with a 0.035-in. (0.089-cm) Kirschner wire placed along the radial border of the scaphoid perpendicular to the plane of the fracture 9.

Fluoroscopy was used to confirm the reduction of the fracture and placement of the wire.

A guide wire for the cannulated screw was inserted parallel to the K-wire. Its position was verified under fluoroscopy. It was overdrilled and taped. An appropriate length cannulated Herbert screw was inserted from distal to proximal over the guide wire that was then removed.

The first Kirschner wire edge was left in place with its edge in subcutaneous tissue for easy removal after 8 weeks.

After thorough irrigation, repair of the long radiolunate and radioscaphocapitate ligaments was done. The wound was closed in layers: the subcutaneous tissue with vicryl 3.0 and skin with monocryl 4.0 in subcuticular fashion.

A sterile dressing was applied. Tourniquet was deflated. A thumb spica cast was applied.

The patient was transferred to the recovery room.

Dr. Staff Attending Surgeon was present, scrubbed, and participated actively in all aspects of the procedure.

Chapter 92
Volar Ganglion Excision

Anthony V. Mollano, M.D.

COMMON INDICATIONS
- Unsightly or painful ganglion
- Interference with function
- Refractory to conservative therapy, from needle aspiration to steroid injection

POSSIBLE COMPLICATIONS
- Neurovascular damage, including radial artery injury
- Recurrence 5 %

ESSENTIAL STEPS
1. Administer anesthesia
2. Exsanguinate arm and inflate tourniquet
3. Perform volar wrist 1.5 cm transverse incision over ganglion
4. Dissect down to cyst, avoiding vigorous retraction to protect nearby nerves, tendons, and vessels
5. Amputate both cyst and its stalk (minimizes recurrence risk) adjacent to flexor carpi radialis tendon; if ganglion envelopes the radial artery, leave a small piece of cyst wall on the artery, and do not peel the entire lesion off the artery
6. Irrigate wound, deflate tourniquet, close skin with 5-0 nylon, and apply short-arm plaster splint

S. Saghieh et al. (eds.), *Operative Dictations in Orthopedic Surgery*,
DOI 10.1007/978-1-4614-7479-1_92,
© Springer Science+Business Media New York 2013

OPERATIVE NOTE

Preoperative Diagnosis: Volar wrist ganglion cyst
Procedure: Excision of volar wrist ganglion cyst
Postoperative Diagnosis: Same
Indications: The patient is an X-year-old graduate student who has a volar ganglion cyst that is symptomatic and has caused flexor carpi radialis irritation and tendinitis. Despite conservative treatment, the patient has had no good relief of her symptoms. Patient understood risks and benefits of ganglion excision surgery, and elected to proceed.

Description of Operation: After adequate anesthesia was obtained, the upper extremity was sterilely prepped and draped. The limb was exsanguinated with an Esmarch bandage and tourniquet inflated to 250 mmHg. A volar 1.5 cm transverse incision following one of the distal wrist creases was made directly over the cystic prominence. Careful subcutaneous dissection with tenotomy scissors was done to protect any longitudinal neurovascular structures. The cystic structure just adjacent to the flexor carpi radialis tendon was circumferentially identified. It was amputated at its base overlying the flexor carpi radialis tendon. Its stalk was then followed down to the volar wrist capsule in the radioscaphoid area and elliptically excised and debrided with curette and rongeur. The volar carpal ligaments were identified and were intact. The wound was thoroughly irrigated and the tourniquet deflated after 35 min of total tourniquet time. 5-0 nylon skin closure was performed, followed by application of a padded short-arm plaster splint. Sponge and instrument counts were correct.

Dr. Staff Attending Surgeon was present, scrubbed, and participated actively in all aspects of the procedure.

Chapter 93
Dorsal Ganglion Excision

Said Saghieh, M.D.

COMMON INDICATIONS
- Unsightly or painful ganglion

POSSIBLE COMPLICATIONS
- Infection
- Scar
- Neurologic damage
- Wrist stiffness
- Recurrence 5 %

ESSENTIAL STEPS
1. Dorsal wrist 3 cm transverse incision centered over the ganglion
2. Deep sharp and blunt dissection around the walls of the ganglion
3. Identify the stalk and dissect it free till the level of the scapholunate ligament
4. En bloc excision
5. Skin closure

OPERATIVE NOTE
Preoperative Diagnosis: Dorsal wrist ganglion cyst
Procedure: Excision of dorsal wrist ganglion cyst
Postoperative Diagnosis: Same
Indications: The patient is an ___ year-old m/w who has been complaining of discomfort over his wrist caused by a ganglion cyst.
Description of Operation: After adequate anesthesia was obtained, the upper extremity was sterilely prepped and draped.

S. Saghieh et al. (eds.), *Operative Dictations in Orthopedic Surgery*,
DOI 10.1007/978-1-4614-7479-1_93,
© Springer Science+Business Media New York 2013

The limb was exsanguinated with an Esmarch bandage and tourniquet inflated to 250 mmHg. A 3 cm transverse incision centered over the ganglion was performed. Careful subcutaneous dissection with tenotomy scissors was done to protect any nerve endings. Using blunt and sharp dissection the cyst was detached circumferentially from the surrounding tissues.

The stalk was identified and followed down to the scapholunate ligament. The cyst was shaved off the ligament and excised entirely. The scapholunate ligament and the carpal dorsal capsule were left intact. The wound was thoroughly irrigated and the tourniquet deflated after 35 min of total tourniquet time.

Subcutaneous tissue was closed with vicryl 3.0 and the skin with monocryl in subcuticular fashion. A compressive dressing was applied.

The patient was transferred to the recovery room.

Dr. Staff Attending Surgeon was present, scrubbed, and participated actively in all aspects of the procedure.

Chapter 94
Release de Quervain

Said Saghieh, M.D.

COMMON INDICATIONS
- Pain over the distal styloid of the radius not responding to conservative treatment

POSSIBLE COMPLICATIONS
- Infection
- Incomplete release with persistent pain
- Nerve injury
- Subluxation of the tendons

ESSENTIAL STEPS
1. Oblique incision centered over the first extensor compartment
2. Blunt dissection to protect sensory branches
3. Opening of the tendon sheath
4. Make sure no aberrant tendons
5. Skin closure

OPERATIVE NOTE
Preoperative Diagnosis: De Quervain disease, R/L wrist
Procedure: Release of the first extensor compartment, R/L wrist
Postoperative Diagnosis: Same
Indications: The patient is an X-year-old m/w who has been complaining of pain over the radial styloid. He/she failed conservative treatment including NSAID, bracing, and steroid injection
Description of Operation: The patient was identified in the preoperative holding area and the affected extremity was marked. After adequate anesthesia was obtained, the R/L upper extremity

S. Saghieh et al. (eds.), *Operative Dictations in Orthopedic Surgery*,
DOI 10.1007/978-1-4614-7479-1_94,
© Springer Science+Business Media New York 2013

was sterilely prepped and draped. The limb was exsanguinated with an Esmarch bandage and tourniquet inflated to 250 mmHg.

A 2 cm skin incision that runs from dorsal to volar in a transverse-to-oblique direction, parallel with the skin creases over the area of tenderness in the first dorsal compartment 1 cm proximal to the radial styloid, was made. Careful blunt dissection of the subcutaneous fat was done to protect branches of the superficial radial nerve.

The first extensor compartment tendons (the abductor pollicis longus and the extensor pollicis brevis) were identified proximal to the stenosing dorsal ligament and sheath. The latter was incised to open the first dorsal compartment on its dorsoulnar side.

With the thumb abducted and the wrist flexed, the tendons were freed from their groove. There were no additional or "aberrant" tendons in separate compartments.

The wound was thoroughly irrigated and the tourniquet deflated after 20 min of total tourniquet time.

Subcutaneous tissue was closed with vicryl 3.0 and the skin with monocryl in subcuticular fashion. A compressive dressing was applied.

The patient was transferred to the recovery room.

Dr. _____ was present, scrubbed, and participated actively in all aspects of the procedure.

Part VIII
Hand

Chapter 95
Congenital Trigger Thumb Release

Karim Masrouha, M.D.

COMMON INDICATIONS
- A definitive diagnosis of trigger thumb in a child with the interphalangeal joint in fixed flexion of 20–75°

POSSIBLE COMPLICATIONS
- Infection
- Radial nerve injury
- Adhesions if motion is not begun in the immediate postoperative period

ESSENTIAL STEPS
1. Preoperative assessment (history and physical examination)
2. Incision must be made adjacent to the metacarpophalangeal (MCP) joint crease with the MCP joint in neutral
3. Identify and isolate the digital nerves
4. Use blunt dissection to expose the A1 and C1 pulleys
5. Incise the entire A1 pulley
6. Assess thumb metacarpal extension for any resistance which might require tendon sheath incision
7. Ensure that the skin edges are carefully everted

OPERATIVE NOTE
Preoperative Diagnosis: Congenital Trigger thumb
Procedure: Trigger thumb release
Postoperative Diagnosis: Same
Indications: _____ years old male/female with a trigger thumb diagnosed at birth.

S. Saghieh et al. (eds.), *Operative Dictations in Orthopedic Surgery*,
DOI 10.1007/978-1-4614-7479-1_95,
© Springer Science+Business Media New York 2013

Description of Operation: The patient and surgical site were identified and marked. The patient underwent anesthesia per the anesthesia team. The patient was positioned supine on the operative table. The upper extremity was scrubbed and draped in the standard sterile fashion. A tourniquet was applied to the proximal end of the arm. Using an Esmarch bandage, the upper extremity was fully exsanguinated and the tourniquet was elevated to 180 mmHg.

With the arm in full supination and the thumb held in abduction while keeping the MCP joint in neutral, a transverse skin incision was made adjacent to the MCP joint crease. Skin hooks were then placed on each side of the wound to retract the skin edges. Blunt dissection was performed with blunt-tipped scissors along the axis of the flexor pollicis longus and the fascia beneath the dermis was identified and divided. Using blunt dissection the radial and ulnar proper digital nerves were identified and the A1 and proximal margin of the C1 pulleys were exposed. The skin hooks were then replaced with a right-angle retractor. The flexor pollicis longus was found to have fusiform enlargement. With a surgical blade, the A1 pulley was then completely incised on its radial side, from its proximal to distal margins.

With the MCP joint in the neutral position the interphalangeal joint was brought to full extension without any resistance. The wound was then irrigated and closed with fine, subcutaneous absorbable sutures. The tourniquet was then deflated.

Postoperative regimen: Begin motion immediately. Remove dressing after 48–72 h.

No intraoperative complications.

Staff was present and scrubbed for entire procedure.

Chapter 96

Trigger Finger Release

Karim Masrouha, M.D.

COMMON INDICATIONS

- A definitive diagnosis of trigger finger by history and physical examination, with failure of nonoperative management

POSSIBLE COMPLICATIONS

- Infection
- Incomplete extension
- Persistent trigger finger
- Digital nerve injury
- Bowstringing

ESSENTIAL STEPS

1. Preoperative assessment (history and physical examination)
2. Incision should be made over the metacarpal neck, avoiding the distal palmar crease
3. Identify and avoid the digital nerves adjacent to the flexor tendon
4. Use blunt dissection to expose and identify the demarcation between the A1 and A2 pulleys
5. Release the A1 pulley at the radial side in the second, third, and fourth digits, and on the ulnar side in the fifth digit
6. Release enough of the pulley to allow full extension and range of motion without triggering

S. Saghieh et al. (eds.), *Operative Dictations in Orthopedic Surgery*,
DOI 10.1007/978-1-4614-7479-1_96,
© Springer Science+Business Media New York 2013

OPERATIVE NOTE

Preoperative Diagnosis: Trigger finger
Procedure: Trigger finger release
Postoperative Diagnosis: Same
Indications: _____ year old male/female with trigger finger after failure of nonoperative management
Description of Operation: The patient and surgical site were identified and marked. The patient underwent anesthesia per the anesthesia team. The patient was positioned supine on the operative table. The upper extremity was scrubbed and draped in the standard sterile fashion. A tourniquet was applied to the proximal end of the arm. Using an Esmarch bandage, the upper extremity was fully exsanguinated and the tourniquet was elevated to 250 mmHg.

A transverse 2 cm incision was made over the neck of the affected metacarpal, adjacent to the distal palmar flexion crease. The flexor tendon and sheath were exposed by blunt dissection and division of the subcutaneous tissue and palmar fascia. The A1 and A2 pulleys were identified and the tendon was checked for any pathology. A probe was inserted underneath the A1 pulley which was then released longitudinally until there was full range of motion in the finger without triggering.

The wound was then irrigated and closed with fine, absorbable subcutaneous sutures. The tourniquet was then deflated.

No intraoperative complications.

Staff was present and scrubbed for entire procedure.

Postoperative regimen: Begin motion immediately. Remove dressing after 48–72 h.

Chapter 97
Flexor Tendon Repair

Saad Dibo, M.D. and Joseph Bakhach, M.D.

COMMON INDICATIONS
- Traumatic laceration/rupture of flexor tendon
- Spontaneous rupture of flexor tendon

POSSIBLE COMPLICATIONS
- Infection
- Scar
- Adhesions
- Rupture of repair
- Flexion contractures
- Wound dehiscence

ESSENTIAL STEPS
1. Prep and drape affected extremity
2. Tourniquet placement
3. Generous extensile incision oriented obliquely between finger creases
4. Extension of incision/wound to identify tendon stumps
5. Cruciate pulleys opened as necessary, preservation of annular pulleys
6. Retrieval of tendon stump
7. Placement of core sutures
8. Approximation of tendon ends
9. Epitendinous repair
10. Wound closure
11. Proper splint placement

S. Saghieh et al. (eds.), *Operative Dictations in Orthopedic Surgery*,
DOI 10.1007/978-1-4614-7479-1_97,
© Springer Science+Business Media New York 2013

OPERATIVE NOTE

Preoperative Diagnosis: Flexor tendon rupture (specify the traumatic etiology if possible, the level of skin injury, and the shape of the finger when the injury happened)

Procedure: Repair of flexor tendon rupture of the (specify which one if possible)

Postoperative Diagnosis: Same

Indications: __ yo female/male who sustained an injury (specify type and time of injury) to their hand/wrist/finger resulting in transection of the flexor tendon (specify finger or which tendon, the level of injury, the quality of the skin (presence of skin defect/laceration/clean cut) as diagnosed by the preoperative examination).

Or ___ yo female/male who suffered spontaneous rupture of flexor tendon (usually secondary to RA).

Description of Operation: The patient and operative site were identified and marked. He/she was brought into the operative suite and placed supine on the operating table. The patient was induced into general endotracheal anesthesia without difficulty/ or the patient underwent regional block of the involved extremity. IV antibiotics were administered. A tourniquet over soft-roll was placed over the injured extremity.

The patient was prepped and draped in the usual sterile fashion. The extremity was exsanguinated with an Esmark and the tourniquet was inflated to 250 mm of mercury.

(If the wound edges are not clean and need debridement) The wound edges were debrided and freshened using a sharp number 15 blade. The area of the injury was explored for evidence of the tendon stumps, but the stumps were not visible in the wound. The incision was extended in a Bruner zigzag fashion. The two neurovascular bundles were exposed and protected.

Zone I injury (Zone I = flexor digitorum profundus (FDP) insertion to distal tip)

The C3 and C4 cruciate were opened in order to find the proximal FDP stump. Care was taken to spare the A4 and A5 pulleys. The proximal stump of the FDP tendon was gently pulled out from the flexor fibrous tube and held in place by a 25-gauge needle passed transversely through the tendon and pulley apparatus.

If enough tendon remains distally:

The two ends of the tendon were approximated using a ____ stitch with a ____ suture using modified Kessler or Becker MGH four-strand repair.

If the distal stump of the tendon is not large enough to accept a suture repair:

A periosteal flap was created at the former insertion site of the tendon on the distal phalanx. A drill was used to create an oblique hole through the proximal distal phalanx from the palmar aspect through fingernail distal to the lunula. A double armed 3-0 suture was placed through the tendon stump and passed through the bone hole. The sutures were passed through a cotton-padded button placed over the fingernail and tied in place.

Additional peripheral 6-0 prolene sutures were taken to the periosteum. The tourniquet was released and hemostasis was obtained. The incisions were closed with .... sutures.

Zone II injury (Zone II = origin of flexor tendon sheath to insertion of superficialis tendon over the midportion of the middle phalanx)

The original incision was extended proximally and distally in a zigzag fashion (or midlateral incisions) to identify tendon stumps. The digital artery and nerve were identified and protected. Exposure of the contents of the sheath was done by opening the C2 cruciate pulley obliquely and reflecting laterally the two flaps of sheath located between the distal edge of the A2 pulley and the proximal edge of the A4 pulley. Distally, the two slips of the FDS tendon were identified and prepared. Flexion of the PIP and DIP delivered the FDP tendon stump into the cruciate pulley window.

Alternatively ... method of Sourmelis and McGrouther (in case the proximal stumps of the FDS and FDP tendons are retracted to the palm).

A small plastic catheter (infant NG tube) was passed from the site of injury proximally through the flexor tendon sheath. A 1 cm incision was made at the level of the distal palmar crease proximal to the A1 pulley. The catheter was sutured to both tendons at this level. The plastic catheter was then pulled distally to deliver the tendon stumps through the flexor tendon sheath into the cruciate pulley window. The palmar wound is closed using ... skin sutures.

Alternatively ... method of Morris and Martin

The tendon stump was visible within the flexor sheath, but not retrievable with non-toothed forceps. A small skin hook was passed through the flexor sheath to the level of the tendon stumps. The hook was then used to engage the tendon and draw it into the cruciate window.

Following delivery of the proximal and distal stumps, a 25-gauge needle was passed transversely through the tendon sheath and tendons to secure the stumps in place. The proper anatomic relationship of the FDS and FDP tendons proximally and at the decussation of the FDS slips and the chiasm of Camper, as well as within the fibroosseous pulley system was reestablished before repair. Core sutures were placed in all tendon stumps (proximal and distal FDP and FDS slips). The tendon stumps were approximated (specify what technique: Modified Kessler or other, and what suture). An epitendinous repair was performed using a ___ suture in a ____ stitch. The flexor tendon sheath was left open to spontaneous healing.

The tourniquet was released and hemostasis was obtained. The wounds were closed using .... sutures.

The patient was placed in a large bulky dressing with the wrist in midflexion, the MCP join in full flexion, and the PIP and DIP joints in full extension.

Tourniquet time was .... minutes.

No immediate complications.

Dr. .... was present and scrubbed for the entire procedure.

Chapter 98
Extensor Repair

Firas Kawtharani, M.D.

COMMON INDICATIONS
- Rupture of extensor tendon, dorsum of hand

POSSIBLE COMPLICATIONS
- Infection
- Scar
- Adhesions
- Rupture of repair

ESSENTIAL STEPS
1. Extension of incision/wound to identify tendon stumps
2. Suturing the tendon
3. Proper splint placement

OPERATIVE NOTE

Preoperative Diagnosis: Acute extensor tendon transection, — finger, R/L hand

Procedure: Primary repair of extensor tendon transection (2–5 finger), R/L hand

Postoperative Diagnosis: Same

Indications: __ yo female/male who sustained an injury to the dorsum of the r/l hand resulting in transection of the extensor tendon.

Description of Operation: The patient and the surgical site were correctly identified. The patient was placed in the supine position on the operating table with the involved extremity on a hand table. A tourniquet was placed over soft roll on the affected upper

S. Saghieh et al. (eds.), *Operative Dictations in Orthopedic Surgery*,
DOI 10.1007/978-1-4614-7479-1_98,
© Springer Science+Business Media New York 2013

extremity. IV antibiotics were administered. Regional anesthesia was initiated by the anesthesia team without difficulty. The extremity was prepped and draped in the usual sterile fashion. It was exsanguinated with an Esmark and the tourniquet was inflated to 250 mmHg. The area of the injury was explored for evidence of the tendon stumps, but the stumps were not visible in the wound. The incision was extended in a zigzag fashion.

The ruptured extensor tendon was identified, the two edges approximated and sutured with a nonabsorbable 4.0 ticron in a modified Kessler fashion. The skin was closed with interrupted 5-0 nylon sutures.

A compressive dressing was applied. The repair was protected with a volar splint with the wrist in extension. The tourniquet was deflated.

Staff was present for the entire procedure.

Chapter 99

CMC Ligament Reconstruction and Tendon Interposition

Aru El Khatib, M.D. and Joseph Bakhach, M.D.

COMMON INDICATIONS

- OA of the trapezio-metacarpal joint (thumb CMC), with or without involvement of the trapezio-scaphoid joint, manifested by persistent pain after failure of conservative management

POSSIBLE COMPLICATIONS

- Wound infection/dehiscence
- Neuroma and neuropathies due to injury to superficial radial nerve branches during dissection
- Diminished pinch strength
- Loss of carpal–metacarpal alignment postoperatively
- Rare: complex regional pain syndrome

ESSENTIAL STEPS

1. Incision of skin
2. Identification and preservation/mobilization of superficial radial nerve branches and radial artery
3. Arthrotomy of CMC and scaphotrapezial joints
4. Resection of trapezium in entirety (pantrapezial arthrosis) or just the distal portion (only trapezio-metacarpal involvement)—care taken to preserve FCR tendon deep
5. Fashioning slide hole in metacarpal
6. Raising flap of FCR—passing through hole
7. Positioning and pinning of thumb

S. Saghieh et al. (eds.), *Operative Dictations in Orthopedic Surgery*,
DOI 10.1007/978-1-4614-7479-1_99,
© Springer Science+Business Media New York 2013

8. Placing and suture anchoring of the tendon flap
9. Repair of the capsule
10. Irrigation and closure
11. Cast/splint placement

OPERATIVE REPORT

Preoperative Diagnosis: Pantrapezial arthrosis R/L thumb, or of only the trapezio-metacarpal joint

Procedure: Trapezium resection, ligament reconstruction, and tendon interposition arthroplasty of left thumb

Postoperative Diagnosis: Same

Indications: ___y.o. M/F with long-standing history of pain at the base of the R/L thumb. Failing conservative treatments, and showing significant findings of degeneration on XR. After explanation of risks and benefits, and answering of all questions, the patient elected to proceed with surgical management and informed consent was obtained.

Description of Operation: The patient was identified by anesthesia in the pre-op area and brought to the operating room. Patient was placed in a supine position on the operating table and all pressure points were padded. The R/L upper extremity was extended onto an arm board. After the induction of satisfactory general anesthesia, the R/L upper extremity was prepped and draped in the usual fashion. The limb was then exsanguinated with an Esmarch bandage and the tourniquet, which had previously been applied about the proximal arm over abundant Sof-Rol padding, was inflated to ___ mmHg.

A chevron-shaped incision was then made centered over the dorsum of the CMC joint of the R/L thumb. Subcutaneous tissues were bluntly separated. Small branches of the superficial radial nerve were identified and protected. The skin flap was then suture-retracted. The fascia overlying the dorsal branch of the radial artery was incised. The radial artery was mobilized and small branches were cauterized using electrocautery. It was gently retracted with a vessel loop. The first dorsal wrist compartment tendons were retracted radially.

A longitudinal arthrotomy was then made in the scaphotrapezial and carpometacarpal joints. Dorsal and palmar capsular flaps were elevated as far as the trapeziotrapezoid joint and the radial margin of the trapezium.

All cartilage had been eroded from the base of the thumb metacarpal as well as the trapezial articular surface. Proximally, there was thinning of cartilage at the scaphotrapezial joint. A Lempert rongeur was then used to remove the trapezium in its entirety piecemeal. The FCR tendon was left intact and mobilized.

A 0.062 Kirschner wire was then used to make a pilot hole from the dorsal cortex of the thumb metacarpal, exiting the intramedullary canal just dorsal to the volar beak. This was enlarged with a 2.4 mm burr.

A ____suture was pre-placed at the insertion of the FCR tendon into the base of the index metacarpal. A looped wire was then passed through the canal that had previously been fashioned in the thumb metacarpal shaft.

A distally based flap of FCR tendon encompassing one-half the circumference of the tendon and measuring approximately ___ cm in length was then raised through three small volar forearm incisions. This tendon was then passed through the intramedullary canal hole previously described in the thumb metacarpal using the looped wire. The tendon was then passed around the remaining intact portion of the FCR tendon.

The thumb was then placed in maximum extension and abduction with care taken to preserve space of an approximate size equal to the resected trapezium. It was then pinned into this position using a 0.062 Kirschner wire passed from the thumb metacarpal into the hand. This wire was bent over outside the skin and cut.

The wounds were irrigated with sterile saline solution. With the wrist in slight flexion and gentle tension on the distally based tendon flap, the previously placed ____ suture was used to anchor this tendon weave to the intact portion of the FCR tendon. Multiple additional _____ sutures were placed at this level.

The remaining tail of FCR tendon was then placed in the space created by trapezium resection to act as an interpositional arthroplasty. The dorsal capsule was then closed using multiple sutures of _____, taking care that certain capsule was closed to the capsule adjacent to the scaphoid bone as well as to incorporate the tendon weave over the dorsum of the thumb metacarpal.

The tourniquet was deflated and bleeding was controlled with compression and electrocautery. Irrigation was completed for all wounds. All wounds were then closed using ____ sutures applied in interrupted simple fashion. Xeroform was wrapped about the base of the pin. A dry sterile dressing was applied which consisted of ____, and a short-arm thumb spica splint.

The tourniquet inflation time was ____ and the deflation time was ____, for a total time of ___ minutes.

The patient was awakened, extubated and taken to the PACU in stable condition.

Chapter 100

Carpal Tunnel Release: Open Technique

Karim Masrouha, MD

COMMON INDICATIONS

- An established diagnosis of carpal tunnel syndrome based on clinical history and physical findings with diagnostic electrophysiologic studies

POSSIBLE COMPLICATIONS

- Transection of the palmar cutaneous branch of the median nerve, the palmar arch, the main trunk of the median nerve, the recurrent motor branch of the median nerve
- Adherence of the median nerve to the flexor tendons and the skin
- Flexor tendon bowstringing
- Wound hematoma
- Infection

ESSENTIAL STEPS

1. Preoperative assessment (history and physical examination)
2. Care must be made to avoid the palmar sensory branch of the median nerve when extending the incision (if severed, section it at its origin)
3. Use blunt dissection of the deep fascia
4. When dissecting the transverse carpal ligament avoid the median nerve and its recurrent branch and extend the dissection to its distal end, which may be farther than expected
5. Release all components of the flexor retinaculum
6. Irrigate the wound and close only the skin

S. Saghieh et al. (eds.), *Operative Dictations in Orthopedic Surgery*,
DOI 10.1007/978-1-4614-7479-1_100,
© Springer Science+Business Media New York 2013

OPERATIVE NOTE

Preoperative Diagnosis: Carpal tunnel syndrome
Procedure: Carpal tunnel release: Open technique
Post-op Diagnosis: Same
Indications: _____ year old male/female with a _____ month history of pain, numbness, and paresthesias along the distribution of the medial nerve distal to the wrist and failure of nonoperative management.

Description of Operation: The patient and surgical site were identified and marked. The patient underwent anesthesia per the anesthesia team. The patient was positioned supine on the operative table. A tourniquet was applied and the arm was placed on a hand table with the forearm fully supinated. The upper extremity was scrubbed and draped in the standard sterile fashion. Using an Esmarch bandage, the upper extremity was fully exsanguinated and the tourniquet was elevated to 250 mmHg.

A 3 cm skin incision starting at the distal wrist crease was made just ulnar to and parallel with the thenar crease. The incision was deepened through the subcutaneous tissue. Under $2.5 \times$ loupe magnification, sharp dissection was carried down to the superficial palmar fascia, which was divided longitudinally. The transverse carpal ligament was exposed. Its proximal edge was isolated at the level of the distal palmar crease and incised longitudinally with a scalpel in line with the ring finger ray and medial to the thenar muscles.

The median nerve was identified. A blunt dissector was inserted between the nerve and the distal part of the transverse carpal ligament. The latter was divided using a scalpel.

The proximal edge of the incision was elevated with skin hooks and the antebrachial fascia divided for 2 cm proximal to the wrist crease along the ring finger axis.

The wound was then irrigated and the tourniquet was deflated. Hemostasis was obtained.

The skin was closed with 4-0 nylon mattress sutures.

A sterile dressing and an elastic bandage were applied.

No intra-operative complications.

Staff was present and scrubbed for entire procedure.

Postoperative regimen: The bandage is to be kept for 2 weeks. Avoid dependent positioning. Immediate use of hand with gradual resumption to normal daily use is encouraged.

Chapter 101
Digital Nerve Epineurial Repair

Saad Dibo, M.D. and Ghassan S. Abu-Sittah, M.B.Ch.B., F.R.C.S.

COMMON INDICATIONS

- Acute or subacute repair of nerve injury (Sunderland's classifications: fourth or fifth degree injury to nerves)

POSSIBLE COMPLICATIONS

- Persistent paresthesias or dysesthesias
- Infection
- Scar/contracture
- Neuroma formation

ESSENTIAL STEPS

1. Prep and drape affected extremity and one or both lower extremities for possible harvesting of nerve graft
2. Tourniquet to each extremity
3. Generous extensile incision
4. Exposure and mobilization of nerve (work from normal to injured area) using jeweler's forceps with gentle handling (use 2 or 3 times magnification)
5. Preparation of nerve ends
6. Identification and avoidance of adjacent digital artery injury
7. Orientation and assessment of tension of nerve ends
8. Epineurial repair using 9-0 or 8-0 nylon using minimal amount of sutures necessary to appose the entire epineurium on the anterior site and the posterior side
9. Wound closure and splinting

S. Saghieh et al. (eds.), *Operative Dictations in Orthopedic Surgery*,
DOI 10.1007/978-1-4614-7479-1_101,
© Springer Science+Business Media New York 2013

OPERATIVE NOTE

Preoperative Diagnosis: Acute or subacute digital nerve injury following (specify type and time of trauma)

Procedure: Digital nerve exploration and epineurial repair

Postoperative Diagnosis: Same

Indications: ____ yo male or female sustaining complete or partial transection injury to digital nerve. Risks and benefits of digital nerve exploration and repair were discussed with the patient.

Description of Operation: The patient and operative site were identified and marked. He/she was brought into the operative suite and placed supine on the operating table. The patient was induced into general endotracheal anesthesia without difficulty/ or the patient underwent regional block of the involved extremity. IV antibiotics were administered. A tourniquet over soft-roll was placed over the injured extremity. The tourniquet was placed up to 250 mm of mercury.

The injured extremity and one leg was prepped and draped in the usual sterile fashion. A Bruner zigzag incision was performed under loop magnification and tourniquet control. Normal nerve was identified in an unscarred tissue bed both proximally and distally and dissection continued toward the zone of injury. The adjacent digital artery was identified, dissected, and protected (the digital artery was found to be injured and was repaired, or was ligated because repair was not possible, after insuring that finger perfusion was not compromised preoperatively). The neuroma of the proximal stump and glioma of the distal stump were resected sharply with a single-edged razor over a moistened wooden tongue depressor or sharp blade. A single 8-0 epineural suture was placed to determine tension. Epineural interrupted suturing was then performed with 8-0 (or 9-0) monofilament prolene on 70–130 μm taper point needle. Nerve edges were sutured circumferentially in appropriate alignment and tightened without bunching the epineurium. Nerve repair was achieved under no tension during finger extension. Wound was irrigated and closed with ... sutures. The tourniquet was released following application of the dressing and finger splint. The patient was extubated in the operative suite and taken to the recovery room in stable condition.

Tourniquet time was .... minutes.

No immediate complications.

Dr. .... was present and scrubbed for the entire procedure.

Chapter 102

Swan Neck Deformity Reconstruction: Flexor Digitorum Superficialis PIP Tenodesis

Saad Dibo, M.D. and Bishara Atiyeh, M.D., F.A.C.S.

COMMON INDICATIONS
- Cosmetically or functionally symptomatic hyperextension of the proximal interphalangeal (PIP) joint and flexion of the distal interphalangeal joint often associated with rheumatoid arthritis

POSSIBLE COMPLICATIONS
- Infection
- Wound contracture
- Relapse of finger deformity

ESSENTIAL STEPS
1. Prep and drape the affected extremity
2. Application of tourniquet
3. Bruner type of incision
4. Midline dissection extension to protect the neurovascular bundle
5. Partial transverse incision on the lateral aspect of the flexor tendon sheath adjacent to the A3 pulley
6. Identification of the lateral slip of the FDS tendon
7. Transection of the lateral FDS slip 10 mm proximal to the insertion on the middle phalynx

S. Saghieh et al. (eds.), *Operative Dictations in Orthopedic Surgery*,
DOI 10.1007/978-1-4614-7479-1_102,

8. Suture the distal-based lateral FDS slip to the ipsilateral aspect of the proximal phalynx including the periosteum and the base of Cleland's/Grayson's ligaments with the PIP joint held in 30° flexion
9. Ensure the proximal FDS and the FDP are moving freely after the repair
10. Repair the partial transverse incision in the flexor tendon sheath
11. Wound closure and dorsal block extension splint

OPERATIVE REPORT

Preoperative Diagnosis: Swan Neck deformity (specify finger)

Procedure: Correction of Swan Neck deformity of the ... finger

Postoperative Diagnosis: Same

Indications: This is a ----year-old lady/man with rheumatoid arthritis, who presents with a swan neck deformity of the ---- finger.

Description of Operation: The patient and operative site were identified and marked. He/she was brought into the operative suite and placed supine on the operating table. The patient was induced into general endotracheal anesthesia without difficulty/ or the patient underwent regional block of the involved extremity. IV antibiotics were administered. A tourniquet over soft-roll was placed over the injured extremity.

The patient was prepped and draped in the usual sterile fashion. The extremity was exsanguinated with an Esmark bandage and the tourniquet was inflated to 250 mm of mercury.

The skin was incised along the preoperative markings with a 15 blade, and the subcutaneous tissue was dissected in the mid-axial plane to the level of the flexor tendon sheath. Care was taken to prevent injury to the flexor tendon sheath and pulley system. Subcutaneous tissue dissection was extended ulnarly until the ulnar digital nerve and artery were identified. These were then retracted ulnar-ward to visualize Cleland's ligament and the ulnar portion of the flexor tendon sheath. The A3 pulley was identified, and a transverse incision extending from the mid-axial plane to the ulnar margin of the flexor tendon sheath was created to retrieve the ulnar slip of the FDS tendon just proximal to its insertion on the middle phalanx. Separation between the FDS tendon slips was extended proximally then cut transversely to harvest an 8–10 mm segment of the distal most portion of the ulnar FDS slip, maintaining its distal attachment on the middle phalynx. The proximal end of the distal ulnar FDS stump was then rotated dorsally and sutured to the periosteum of the ulnar aspect of the proximal phalanx, as well as Cleland's ligament, using 4-0 nonabsorbable braided suture in a locking fashion while holding the finger PIP in 30° of flexion. Excursion of the residual proximal FDS slip, as well as the FDP, was confirmed after this repair to ensure these remaining tendons were free. The PIP joint was then gently extended passively to ensure that the performed tenodesis prevented hyperextension.

The transverse incision of the flexor tendon sheath was repaired with .... sutures.

The wound was copiously irrigated with normal saline, and ... sutures were used to close the skin. A sterile dressing was applied, followed by extension block splint with an ulnar strut, and the tourniquet was released. The patient was transferred to recovery in stable condition.

Dr. .... was present and scrubbed for the entire procedure.

Chapter 103

Boutonnière Deformity: PIP Joint Arthroplasty

Erin E. Forest, M.D.

COMMON INDICATIONS
- Boutonnière deformity secondary to rheumatoid arthritis causing significant pain
- Proximal interphalangeal joint (PIP) joint arthroplasty is also sometimes used in cases of severe osteoarthritis

POSSIBLE COMPLICATIONS
- Prosthetic failure, loosening or migration
- Recurrence of deviation deformity
- Erosion of prosthesis through the skin
- Infection

ESSENTIAL STEPS
1. Inflation of tourniquet
2. Incision of the extensor mechanism
3. Resection of the proximal phalanx condyles
4. Broaching of the endosteal cavities
5. Sizing and placement of the prosthesis
6. Closure of the extensor mechanism and skin
7. Dressing and splinting of finger in full extension

OPERATIVE NOTE
Preoperative Diagnosis: PIP rheumatoid arthritis
Procedure: PIP joint arthroplasty
Postoperative Diagnosis: Same

S. Saghieh et al. (eds.), *Operative Dictations in Orthopedic Surgery*,
DOI 10.1007/978-1-4614-7479-1_103,
© Springer Science+Business Media New York 2013

Indications: The patient is a ____ year old male/female with Boutonnière deformity of the PIP joint of the ____ finger secondary to rheumatoid arthritis and causing debilitating pain.

Description of Operation: Implants Used:

The patient was brought back to the operating room and placed in the supine position. Regional anesthesia was performed by the anesthesia team. The patient was given antibiotics for perioperative prophylaxis. A well-padded tourniquet was placed on the ____ upper extremity. The ____ upper extremity was then prepped and draped in the usual sterile fashion.

The limb was exsanguinated and the tourniquet inflated to ____ mmHg. Skin incision was made over the dorsal surface of the ____ finger at the level of the PIP joint. A subcutaneous flap was raised radially and ulnarly, to expose the capsule and the extensor mechanism. A distally based, rectangular-shaped flap at the extensor mechanism was made, to allow exposure of the joint. An awl was used to enter the canal of the proximal phalanx. Then the alignment awl was placed. This was used to line up the cutting guide for the end of the proximal phalanx. This cut was then made distal to the collateral ligaments, with care taken not to damage them.

We then broached to a number _____. The cutting guide was then used to make the oblique volar cut. We put in the size ____ trial component and it fit well and had good alignment. A burr was then used to open up the canal on the proximal aspect of the middle phalanx, which was then broached to a size ____. Both trial components were then placed, and the joint had good stability and good motion, including full extension.

The wound was irrigated. The permanent components were then placed. The joint did not subluxate or dislocate with motion and had good stability and motion. The tourniquet was then deflated. The extensor mechanism was closed with four figure-of-eight, 3-0 Ethibond sutures. The skin was closed with 5-0 nylon sutures. We again checked the stability and range of motion and it was satisfactory. We took intraoperative plain films, to check position of the implants, and they were satisfactory.

The patient was placed in a splint, in extension. The patient was transported back to the recovery room in satisfactory condition.

Tourniquet time:

Postoperative activity restrictions: Extension splint for 7–10 days, then a removable splint. Gentle ROM exercises beginning at 2 weeks postoperatively.

No intraoperative complications.

Faculty was present and scrubbed for the entire case.

Chapter 104

Open Reduction and Internal Fixation of Unicondylar Phalangeal Fractures: Screw Fixation

Ziad Elkhoury, M.D.

COMMON INDICATIONS
- Displaced unicondylar fractures (1 mm or more)
- Open unicondylar fractures
- Non-displaced unicondylar fractures, which are all inherently unstable (relative indication)

POSSIBLE COMPLICATIONS
- Damage to the neurovascular structures (lateral approach only)
- Infection (higher incidence when K wires are used)
- Fixation failure
- PIP joint stiffness
- DIP joint stiffness (rare)
- Late post-traumatic arthritis (incidence unknown)

ESSENTIAL STEPS
1. A mid-axial or lateral skin incision (for large fragments with no articular comminution). A dorsal longitudinal midline incision (for comminuted fractures)
2. Release of Cleland's ligament (lateral approach). Splitting the extensor tendon (dorsal approach)
3. Joint debridement and bone grafting when needed (for comminuted fractures only)
4. Fracture reduction
5. Screw application with countersinking of the head

S. Saghieh et al. (eds.), *Operative Dictations in Orthopedic Surgery*,
DOI 10.1007/978-1-4614-7479-1_104,
© Springer Science+Business Media New York 2013

6. Wound irrigation
7. Tendon closure (dorsal approach only)
8. Skin closure
9. Application of bulky dressing

NOTE THESE VARIATIONS

Noncomminuted vs. comminuted fractures requiring lateral or dorsal approach, respectively

Bone grafting for comminuted fractures when required

Augmentation of fixation with a K wire when required

OPERATIVE NOTES

Preoperative Diagnosis: Unicondylar phalanx fracture

Procedure: Open reduction screw fixation of a unicondylar phalanx fracture

Postoperative Diagnosis: Same

Indications: This ___ years old male/female presented with a [FRACTURE DESCRIPTION] unicondylar fracture of the left/right [SPECIFY DIGIT] proximal phalanx. Open reduction internal fixation using screws/screws and K wire was indicated

Description of Operation: The patient was placed in the supine position, the left/right upper extremity was placed on an arm board. All bony prominences were padded. A pneumatic tourniquet was applied over soft roll around the left/right upper extremity. Regional anesthesia was initiated without complication. Time out was performed. The surgical site was prepped and draped in the usual sterile manner. The limb was exsanguinated with an Emarch and the tourniquet was inflated.

A 3 cm lateral incision was made over the PIP joint of the [AFFECTED] finger starting 2 cm proximal to the interphalangeal flexion crease and ending 1 cm distal to it. The subcutaneous tissue was dissected. Cleland's ligament was released and the extensor hood mechanism was retracted dorsally. The volar neurovascular bundle was identified and gently retracted volarly throughout the procedure. The fracture was reduced and hold temporary with a baby bone clamp.

Using lag technique and overdrilling of the near cortex, a 1.5 mm miniscrew was introduced proximal to the origin of the collateral ligament, from the fracture fragment into the proximal phalangeal shaft.

The head of the screw was countersunk. Using the same technique, a second screw was introduced proximal to the first across the fracture line.

[If the fragment is too small to hold two screws: A K wire was introduced proximal to the screw across the fracture line, and cut flush with the bony surface.]

Fluoroscopy was used to confirm adequate fixation.

The wound was irrigated with normal saline. The skin was closed with interrupted horizontal mattress 5-0 nylon sutures. A sterile bulky bandage was applied. The tourniquet was deflated.

The patient tolerated the procedure well with no complications.

A staff was present and scrubbed during the whole procedure.

Chapter 105
Tendon Transfers for Radial Nerve Palsy

Mark L. Hagy, M.D.

COMMON INDICATIONS
- Radial nerve palsy providing the patient with the ability to extend the wrist
- Metacarpophalangeal joint extension
- Combination of thumb extension and abduction

POSSIBLE COMPLICATIONS
- Infection
- Tendon rupture
- Limited wrist or digital motion

ESSENTIAL STEPS
1. Incision over the FCU
2. FCU harvested and freed of adhesions
3. Incision distal to medial epicondyle
4. FCU freed proximally
5. Incision made over PT insertion
6. Subperiosteal release of PT at its insertion
7. PT transfer to ECRB
8. FCU transfer to EDC 2-5
9. EPL and PL harvest from previous incisions
10. PL transfer to EPL

S. Saghieh et al. (eds.), *Operative Dictations in Orthopedic Surgery*,
DOI 10.1007/978-1-4614-7479-1_105,
© Springer Science+Business Media New York 2013

OPERATIVE NOTE

Preoperative Diagnosis: Radial nerve palsy
Procedure: Flexor to extensors tendon transfer
Postoperative Diagnosis: Radial nerve palsy
Description of Operation: The patient is identified in the pre-op holding area and brought to the room. Ancef 1 g is given preoperatively. The patient is placed supine on the operating room table. Arm is placed on a hand table. Soft roll followed by tourniquet is applied to the proximal aspect of the arm. The extremity is prepped and draped in a sterile fashion. The tourniquet is turned up.

A longitudinal incision is made over the FCU tendon in distal half of the forearm. The distal limb of the incision is J-shaped, with the transverse limb being long enough to reach the PL tendon. The FCU tendon is identified and transected just proximal to its insertion onto the pisiform. The tendon is freed up as far proximally as the incision will allow. A tendon stripper is used to free the tendon of all adhesion to within a few centimeters of its origin. At this point, generous debridement of the muscle belly is carried out to facilitate cosmetic appearance for the transfer.

A second incision is made 4 cm below the medial epicondyle and angles across the dorsum of the proximal forearm aiming for Lister's tubercle. The deep fascia overlying the FCU muscle belly is further excised. The proximal extent of the muscle is completely freed. The most proximal aspect of the muscle is avoided to prevent denervation of the musculature.

A third incision is made on the volar-radial aspect of the midforearm, beginning in the area of PT insertion and angling back on the dorsum of the distal forearm towards Lister's tubercle. The tendon of the PT is identified and followed to its insertion. The insertion is released with sharp subperiosteal dissection. The PT is then followed proximally and freed of all adhesions in order to improve excursion. At this juncture the PT tendon and muscle are passed subcutaneously around the radial aspect of the forearm. This was done superficial to brachioradialis (BCR) and extensor carpi radialis longus (ECRL). The insertion is attached into the musculotendinous junction of the ECRB tendon using 3-0. Prior to insertion the wrist is brought into approximately 20–30° of extension in order to establish appropriate tendon tension. Using a tendon passer a pulvertaft tendon weave is carried out 3 times. With each tendon pass the junction between the PT and ECRB is secured with 3-0 vicryl suture.

Subcutaneous dissection is then carried out from the previously made dorsal incision around to the ulnar border of the forearm. At this point a hemostat is used to pull the previously harvested FCU tendon into the dorsal wound. An incision is made in the fascia overlying the EDC tendons just proximal to the extensor retinaculum. The most proximal aspect of the retinaculum is opened. EDC tendons 2-5 are then identified. Again using the tendon passer the FCU tendon is carried through the respective EDC tendon slips. The tendons are opposed using 3-0 vicryl. With attachment of each tendon from index to the ring finger appropriate phalangeal extension is verified. Once appropriate fixation and positioning is verified the EDC tendons proximal to the transfer are cut.

The EPL muscle is then identified in the dorsal wound and divided at its musculotendinous junction. The tendon is then rerouted out of its third dorsal compartment subcutaneously to level of the anatomic snuffbox. The PL tendon is identified in the initial volar incision and transected. The PL tendon is freed up proximally enough to allow a straight-line pull between the PL and rerouted EPL. The PL is delivered following subcutaneous dissection into the dorsal wound. Appropriate tensioning with extension and abduction of the thumb is achieved. A pulvertaft weave is again carried out between these two tendons. The weave is secured with 3-0 vicryl.

The wounds are thoroughly irrigated with saline. Subcutaneous closure is carried out with 2-0 vicryl followed by skin closure with 5-0 nylon. Adaptic, sterile 4×4 gauze is applied followed by soft roll and a volar and dorsal plaster splints. Care is taken to maintain the appropriate positioning of the thumb, wrist, and digits.

The tourniquet is released. The patient is awakened from anesthesia and taken to recovery room without evidence of complication.

Dr._____ was present throughout the entire case.

Part IX
Tumor

Chapter 106

Curettage and Grafting of a Cystic Bone Lesion

Said Saghieh, M.D.

COMMON INDICATIONS
- Unicameral or aneurysmal bone cyst
- Benign bone lesion

POSSIBLE COMPLICATIONS
- Infection
- Recurrence
- Fracture

ESSENTIAL STEPS
1. Skin incision
2. Expose the involved bone
3. Fluoroscopy control
4. Create a window in the cortex
5. Use a curette to scrape the content and the membrane
6. Use adjuvant mechanical or chemical
7. Pack cancellous bone graft into the defect
8. Closure

S. Saghieh et al. (eds.), *Operative Dictations in Orthopedic Surgery*,
DOI 10.1007/978-1-4614-7479-1_106,
© Springer Science+Business Media New York 2013

OPERATIVE NOTE

Preoperative Diagnosis: Unicameral bone cyst of -----, R/L
Procedure: Curettage bone cyst, ----------, bone graft substitute
Postoperative Diagnosis: Same
Indications: This is a —-year-old F/M who presented with acute pain in his/her -------. Radiographs showed evidence of UBC confirmed on CT scan. The cyst did not regress after steroid injection.
Description of Operation: The patient was identified and the affected extremity marked in the preoperative holding area. The patient was taken to the operating room and placed under general anesthesia. Pressure points were padded and the ------ extremity was prepped and draped free. IV antibiotics were administered.

A 5 cm longitudinal skin incision was then made centered over the cystic area as marked with fluoroscopy. Dissection was carried down through the subcutaneous tissue. Fascia was opened. The muscle fibers were split and the bone exposed.

Cobb elevators were used to reflect the periosteum off the bone. Using a 2.5 mm drill bit and fine osteotome, an oblong cortical window 15×8 mm was made. Yellowish clear fluid was discharged from the bone.

A curved curette was inserted and the cyst lining was curetted out and sent to pathology for evaluation. Once the cyst had been thoroughly curetted, a burr was used gently to scrape the walls. Fluoroscopy was used to confirm the extent of the curettage/burring. Next, phenol was injected into the cystic cavity to be washed with 95 % ethanol after few minutes. The cavity was then thoroughly irrigated with normal saline. Cancellous allograft chips (DBM) were then used to pack the cavity.

The periosteal layer was reapproximated with interrupted simple sutures using 2-0 Vicryl. The subcutaneous layer was closed with buried simple sutures using 2-0 Vicryl and the skin closed with a 4-0 Monocryl running stitch in subcuticular fashion.

The patient was awakened from anesthesia and transferred to the recovery room in good conditions.

There was no intraoperative complication.

A staff was present during the procedure.

Chapter 107
Incisional Biopsy: Soft Tissue

Michael J. Huang, M.D.

COMMON INDICATIONS
- Unknown soft-tissue mass—diagnostic and/or therapeutic

POSSIBLE COMPLICATIONS
- Neurologic damage
- Vascular damage
- Incomplete excision
- Wound complications (i.e., infection, dehiscence)

ESSENTIAL STEPS
1. Incision made along mass
2. Subcutaneous dissection
3. Description of what was found
4. Materials sent for pathology and/or microbiology
5. Irrigation, hemostasis, and closure

OPERATIVE NOTE
Preoperative Diagnosis: Mass located ____
Procedure: Incisional biopsy of mass
Postoperative Diagnosis: Same
Indications: __-year-old male/female with a history of a mass located ____.
Description of Operation: The patient was brought to the operating room and placed supine on the operating table. The patient had all pressure points padded and was prepped and draped in a standard surgical fashion. A _ cm long incision was made over the ____ aspect of the mass which was easily palpable. The incision was carried directly down to the lesion which was just beneath the

S. Saghieh et al. (eds.), *Operative Dictations in Orthopedic Surgery*,
DOI 10.1007/978-1-4614-7479-1_107,
© Springer Science+Business Media New York 2013

subcutaneous tissue. The soft tissue mass was identified, and it was dissected from the surrounding tissue. The lesion appeared to be _____ (color, consistency, etc.). Specimens of the tissue were sent to Anatomic Pathology. The tissue and bed of the lesion was cultured for aerobes and anaerobes. After the cultures were taken, a single dose of IV antibiotics was given. The wound was then copiously irrigated and hemostasis was obtained with electrocautery. The wound was closed with 3–0 nylon placed in a vertical mattress fashion. A Xeroform was applied and a sterile dressing was placed. The patient was brought to the recovery room in good condition. There were no complications.

Dr. ____ was present and scrubbed for the entire operation.

A Department of Orthopaedic Surgery faculty member was immediately available for this procedure as documented in the Orthopaedic Department Operating Room Surgeon Backup Schedule.

Chapter 108

Incisional Biopsy: Bone Tumor

Said Saghieh, M.D.

COMMON INDICATIONS
- Bone tumor

POSSIBLE COMPLICATIONS
- Bleeding
- Infection
- Tumor contamination
- Non conclusive specimen

ESSENTIAL STEPS
1. Careful preoperative assessment (history, physical examination, evaluation of imaging studies)
2. Plan skin incision to be included in the definitive resection
3. Go for the most direct approach through the muscle not through intermuscular plan
4. Use fluoroscopy
5. Open cortical window
6. Adequate specimen
7. Hemostasis
8. Closure of the different layers including the muscle
9. Drain if necessary with the exit tract adjacent to the incision
10. Protective weight bearing

S. Saghieh et al. (eds.), *Operative Dictations in Orthopedic Surgery*,
DOI 10.1007/978-1-4614-7479-1_108,
© Springer Science+Business Media New York 2013

OPERATIVE NOTE
Preoperative Diagnosis: Bone tumor
Procedure: Open biopsy
Postoperative Diagnosis: Same
Indications: ___ year-old male/female who was diagnosed with a bone tumor that needs a histologic identification.
Description of Operation: The patient and surgical site were identified and marked. The patient underwent anesthesia per the anesthesia team. The patient was positioned supine on the operative table with all bony prominences padded. IV antibiotics were administered.

Fluoroscopy was used to identify the bone lesion. A 3–5 cm longitudinal skin incision was performed centered over the lesion. The incision was planned to be resected with the tumor at the time of definitive resection. It was deepened through the subcutaneous tissue. The muscle fibers were split down to the periosteum that was incised. With the use of 2.5 mm drill bit, multiple cortical holes were performed in an oval shape. With the use of small-curved osteotome, the cortical window was opened and bone curettage done. A fine metallic suction was used to decrease blood contamination to the surrounding structure.

Closure of the muscle was performed with vicryl 0, subcutaneous tissue with vicryl 2–0 and the skin with monocryl 4–0. A small hemovac was used to drain the wound exiting just proximal to the proximal edge of the wound.

Sterile dressings were applied.

Post-op regimen: Protective-weight bearing for 6 weeks.

No intra-operative complications.

Staff was present and scrubbed for entire procedure.

Index

S. Saghieh et al. (eds.), *Operative Dictations in Orthopedic Surgery*,
DOI 10.1007/978-1-4614-7479-1,
© Springer Science+Business Media New York 2013

Made in the USA
San Bernardino, CA
04 August 2019